# Dyslexia is not a brain disease

# Dyslexia is not a brain disease

*by Rob Christie*

*A guide to what it really is and what we can do about it—for parents, teachers and interested others*

APS Imprint, Fivepin Limited, 91 Crane Street, Salisbury
Wiltshire, SP1 2PU, UK

British Library Cataloguing in Publication Data
A catalogue record for this book is available from the British Library.

© Fivepin  2005
ISBN 1 9038773 9 3

Printed in the United Kingdom by Lightning Source, Milton Keynes

# Contents

# Preface

This book is intended to clear away some of the confusion and mythology surrounding the controversial phenomenon of developmental dyslexia and offer a straightforward guide about what it is and what can be done about it for parents, teachers and interested others.

It is also intended to provide further reading for those who want to know more. For that reason the book is in two parts.

Following the introduction, the first part of the book offers succinct, practical and helpful information about the nature of developmental dyslexia, its causes and what can be done to help those affected by it.

The second part offers more extended information and explanation—sometimes technical—citing research evidence and sources of further reading.

In producing this book, I have drawn on my studies in cognitive neuropsychology and in the various aspects of the English language, and its use as a means of communication, as well as many years of undertaking assessment, recommending remediation for children and adults, and lecturing to a wide range of organisations on the issues.

I hope you will find it interesting and of practical use.

# Part 1

# An introduction to developmental dyslexia

Since dyslexia is dysfunction, disruption or poor development of the facility for communicating in the written form of the language, that is, reading and writing, it should be helpful for the understanding of what it really is and what we can actually do about it to consider in some detail what constitutes reading and what constitutes writing.

For that reason, each of these will be considered in turn, starting with reading—which is traditionally addressed first, although it can be argued that writing and spelling should logically come first, as we shall see later.

But before that we should consider just *why* the deceptively simple but actually very complex activities which comprise the ability to read and write with some facility are so important and their loss or failure to develop to adequate levels so potentially crippling—not least because they are the basis of virtually all human learning.

## The importance of being able to use the written language

Using the written language is a means of communicating information. This is also true of using number. Using the written language allows information which might otherwise be transmitted face to face in the spoken language to be received and reviewed in another time and/or place.

In this modern society, the acquisition and transmission of information in written form for a whole range of social, leisure and occupational purposes are likely to be crucial for most people at some point in their lives. It is therefore crucial for any individual participating in these activities in any way, at any level, for their abilities in this respect to be as good as they can be or as may be required of them.

This applies not only at the 'mechanical' level of reading and writing but also in the highly skilled ability to apply these to the range of register and genre to be found in as many contexts of application as the individual desires or finds necessary (see diagrams on page 6).

For the well-being of individuals in such a society, it is therefore important that any block to satisfactory development of this ability to use the written form of the language or number to appropriate levels should be overcome as quickly and completely as possible. In practice, this means the accurate and complete identification of anything obstructing development of appropriate fluency in these abilities and removal of that blockage wherever possible. This applies to developmental dyslexia as much as anything else.

Using the written language is not a naturally occurring phenomenon. It is a learned facility. If nothing were done to learn it, it would not appear and in societies unlike ours, in which acquisition and transmission of information are largely in written form, that would make little difference to the individual's fundamental ability to make their way in the world.

It is therefore not developmental in the same way as, for example, vision or walking upright are developmental. It is developed rather than develops. It does not evolve by itself. Rather, it is learned, can be taught and improved and fine tuned by formal or informal, intentional or incidental tuition and/or learning.

**Implications for children, young people and all learners: the need for literacy in learning**

It therefore follows that since reading and writing are a means to acquiring and demonstrating possession of the information which forms the basis of every academic subject in education, it is critical that performance in reading and writing is as good as it can be. Without that, access to information and therefore to academic development will be obstructed if not denied.

That means that within formal education, especially in the first few years, development of the skills of reading and communicating in the written form of the language should be the priority—placed above all else—to ensure that poor development of these skills forms no obstruction to learning. This cannot be emphasised too much. All subsequent progress in scholastic learning and in occupation depends on this.

## Implications for adults: the need for functional literacy

For most adults, work is a central part of life. Competence in all occupations, as in all other aspects of life, requires a certain level of ability to acquire information and to communicate information in written form, that is, the ability to read and write. This is called functional literacy by some.

It therefore follows that, since reading and writing are a means to choosing, acquiring, maintaining one's place in and obtaining advancement at appropriate levels in all occupations, and demonstrating possession of the information which forms the basis of all but the most basic jobs, it is critical that performance in reading and writing is as good as it can be or needs to be. Each occupation has its own peculiar demands at appropriate levels. Without that, access to information and therefore to careers development may well be significantly obstructed if not denied.

That means that development of the skills of reading and communicating in the written form of the language should be the priority—placed above all else—to ensure that poor development of these skills forms no obstruction to learning and development. This cannot be emphasised too much. In the modern information-based society, subsequent progress in occupation may depend heavily on it.

Being able to use the written language with facility is empowering and enabling because it is part of every occupation—and more and more, a crucial part. Even routine shift work may require reading production schedules and completing shift handover sheets. Gardening labourers may have to read instructions on pesticide tins and this could be crucial.

It is well known that those who are generally disadvantaged are very often also those who have significant difficulties in literacy and for this reason are even more excluded from social activity in general and occupational access and advancement in particular.

For most people, this is a sensitive issue but it is clearly in their interest for occupational and social inclusion to overcome any difficulties they might have in this respect.

At any given time, there are many persons for whom the possession of these abilities can make the difference between gaining access to, achieving competence in, maintaining or making progress in employment. This is sometimes referred to as having special needs.

Depending on the definition used, anything between 10 per cent and 40 per cent of the population can be said to have some degree of difficulty with reading and/or writing and/or spelling, which may constitute functional illiteracy for the occupation which they seek or in which they work. In some cases, the persons concerned are said to be suffering from something called 'dyslexia' (in fact 'developmental' dyslexia) and this is said to be different from 'ordinary' poor reading or writing in a number of ways and therefore there is a need for special help and/or special treatment.

Whether or not dyslexia, widespread poor reading or writing denies industry access to otherwise competent, and sometimes potentially far more productive, workers and also puts unnecessary strain on the government's employment services' provision by rendering the progress of persons affected inappropriate or ineffective, because of the type of access to employment initiatives and provisions.

The current practices, if any, used for the identification of those demands, and the means of identifying those who fall short of them, vary enormously from place to place and can lead to similar variability, sometimes bordering on the inadequate or ineffectual, in the provision of remedial help.

The complexities of use of the written language are shown below.

## Literacies are complex capabilities

**Literacy and numeracy are vehicles for conveying information**

<u>Range of applications</u>: from most complex to everyday use

Formal, official letters, such as from a solicitor or the council
Argument—pros and cons—requiring a conclusion
Extended narrative—report or novel
Simple narrative—short story or letter

**Requiring...**

Coding and de-coding the spoken language    * EFL/ESOL
Translating—based on meaning

Underpinning skills of writing and reading at base level

**<u>Requiring adequate development of:</u>**

| Skills | Knowledge/Understanding |
|---|---|
| articulating ideas | 'intelligence'/background information |
| spoken form | |

*English as a Foreign Language
English as a Second or Other Language

5

## Literacy and numeracy are complex capabilities which require different levels of skill development

**Level of acquiring information by reading**
- Initial reading skills ('decoding')
  this includes scanning technique, phonological
  awareness and analysis/synthesis skills
- Reading accurately, acquiring information—register and genre*
  from: redundant text, e.g. tabloid newspapers
    semi-redundant text, e.g. quality newspapers
    non-redundant text, e.g. council or solicitor's letters

**Level of communicating in writing**
- Initial writing skills ('encoding')
  this includes handwriting and spelling; subskills
    converting speech to written/typed form (dictation)
    short notes; simple sentences
    pursuit of an argument, complex sentences, embedded clauses
    use of an appropriate register/words and phrasing for the
    purpose

**Level of working with numbers**
- Recognising number, expressing number
- Simple calculations using the four basic operations—accurately
- Complex, multiple operation, calculations—accuracy
- Problem-solving involving interpreting the requirements for the
  resolution of the problem, laying out the structure of the resolution to the
  problem and then solving it

*register approximates to level of complexity
genre approximates to type; e.g. novels or letter-writing or essay

## The nature of reading and communicating in the written form of the language, including spelling

Before embarking on a detailed consideration of what dyslexia is and what we can do about it, understanding it should be helped by understanding what reading and writing are, because dyslexia is about where they go wrong—or fail to develop to the extent expected.

### Reading

1   The ability or skills to acquire or extract information from written or printed text (at least in this context).

*Reading comprehension:* There are other, broader, equally valid meanings such as reading a map or reading the weather signs and even reading a person's attitudes or intentions from the expression on their face).

The assessment of reading ability actually falls into three categories and the tests of these reflect these one or other category, but are more often, wrongly, used interchangeably.

The fundamental aspect of reading is that of reading comprehension. It is sometimes forgotten that there are all kinds of phenomena within this function which aid its performance; for example, the redundancy of the text, the adequacy of concept store (store of 'knowledge' of/familiarity with the subject matter) of the reader for the task and the very complex mental activity of perception of meaning.

2.   The ability to recognise written or printed words.

*Word recognition:* Word recognition is also known as reading 'accuracy'. The results may show, by chance, only some of the words known by the individual but give an estimate on the extent and complexity of the words which they immediately recognise. The set of words which any individual can be expected to recognise is actually specific to that individual and depends on many things such as their experience of their environment for the formation of knowledge of the world around them and especially the words used to describe it and their experience of the words in print. There should be some relationship, but not an exact one, between their word recognition 'vocabulary' and their oral vocabulary.

3. The ability to **identify**—that is, produce a sound version which may or may not be accurate—of written or printed words which are not immediately recognised.

*Word identification (also known as word attack):* This is based on adequate awareness of the phonology—the sound structure—of the spoken language and is usually achieved by application of word identification skills of analysis of a word into syllables, morphemes (part-word) or single sounds (phonemes), then synthesis or 'blending' of these parts into whole words which may then be recognised from their whole word sounds (but sometimes the use of additional knowledge and skills is necessary for this).

Assessment is made on the individual's performance in application of phonological analysis, knowledge of letter/sound relationships—particularly of groups of letters—and then synthesis or 'blending' of these discrete sounds into a unified pattern. The purpose—of which the user must be made aware—of these techniques is to hear and possibly recognise an oral or sound version of a word which is already known to them (already in their oral vocabulary). If the individual does not already possess it in memory in sound form, the pattern produced by analysis and blending in this manner may not be recognised. It is also possible that the correct operation of word identification skills will not produce the usual, and therefore recognisable, sound-form of the word, as for example if the child correctly segments 'canary' into 'can' and 'arry' (rather than 'ayray') which when put together then produces 'cannery', a very different word—and a logical, common mistake.

For a more detailed reading, see page 53.

## Communication in writing or in written form

This is the transmission of information (in the cognitive psychology sense) in the form of the written language (which, in English, uses arbitrary symbols), normally to a receiver in another time or place—so precluding the use of the spoken form. This includes such things as the knowledge of the effects of punctuation and its skilled use, as well as the production of the visual form of words, and is distinct from 'writing' in the literal sense of the physical/motor activity of forming or drawing letter and word-shapes (for a more detailed reading, see page 64).

## Spelling

The ability to produce the 'written'—usually the 'correct'—form of words. This can either be in the context of spontaneous intent to communicate information in the 'written' form of the language or in response to requests to produce specific words presented in a list of spoken words—usually out of their normal context—in the form of 'dictation'.

The 'correct' form or 'spelling' of words in the English language is now often arbitrary for a number of reasons and there are two major routes or strategies for the production of words, that is, spelling. These are known technically as 'addressed spelling' and 'assembled spelling'.

*Addressed spelling* is the form used by skilled spellers until they encounter a word which is not visually familiar to them, at which point they will usually and properly switch to the use of the complementary skill of assembled spelling.

In addressed spelling, the speller knows (has a complete and accurate visual image in permanent memory of) the visual form of the word they are spelling and 'addresses' or accesses that memory store directly when the need arises to write it down. The visual image in memory is then drawn or 'written' (perhaps typed).

*Assembled spelling* is the conversion of the **sound** version of the word stored in permanent memory, bit by bit, into the letters which represent these sounds. During this process, the sound version of the word is apparently held temporarily in 'working' memory (see below).

In assembled spelling, the speller is primarily working on sounds—usually because their 'memory' of the visual form of the word in question is either absent or incomplete—and depending on a range of subskills to help them convert these sounds into letter and word form—frequently resulting in 'phonic' or 'phonetic' spelling where the word is not the 'correct' visual version but, if read aloud, produces the 'correct' original sound.

It also appears that less skilled spellers—those who do not have a large store of the relevant visual images of words—may often use a combination of conversion of the sounds within words together with some half-remembered or poor visual representations of the words, and this can be mutually obstructive when attempts to use the poor visual images interfere with the smooth operation of conversion of the sound form of the word, bit by bit, into the 'written' form.

Unfortunately, in the English language, there is often no fixed relationship even between the 26 letters and the 44 single sounds they are used to represent, although there are many commonly occurring words and part words.

For this reason, assembled spelling is, by its very nature, subject to probability—the likelihood that in **this** word the sounds are represented by **these** letters—perhaps on the basis of use in a similar word which **is** familiar to the speller. It may also require the use of other, complementary techniques. For example, if one didn't know the word, using 'phonics' only might result in the less common word for the branch of a tree, 'bough', being spelled 'bow', because it sounds like the more common word 'how'. Similarly, the 'u' and 'i' letters produce quite different sounds in the words 'fruit', 'build' and 'ruin'. The only real answer to the problem of spelling unfamiliar words is to know what they look like, and that means acquiring and retaining their visual image—usually during the course of reading (for a more detailed reading, see page 65).

Armed with this information, we can now consider reading failure as a result of accident in those who could previously read and write quite well and failure (so far at least) to develop expected* levels of fluency in reading and writing in those who are still learning and/or developing those skills.

## Dyslexia

Developmental dyslexia is a controversial and, for some, very emotive issue. It is said to affect the population to an extent ranging from around 4 per cent to over 25 per cent and its effects are said to be felt in all aspects of life in which reading and writing are in any way important.

Unfortunately, there are many conceptions of what developmental dyslexia is—some much less scientifically tenable than others and some merely a matter of belief—giving rise to a variety of sometimes mutually contradictory perceptions of what, if anything, can be done to minimise or overcome the problems.

Even more confusing is the tendency for some researchers, for example those seeking to prove that certain genes are responsible for difficulty in learning to read, to assume that there is only one conception of developmental dyslexia. Theirs! And these often don't declare what the conception they are working with is. Instead, they apparently assume that there is no controversy about this and go on to 'prove' the hypothesis they are researching without ever considering the validity of its basis.

### The origins and evolution of the concepts of dyslexia

There are in fact two forms of dyslexia: one clearly the result of physical injury and uncontroversial, and the other whose nature, causes and even existence are a matter of dispute.

The first and original form of dyslexia was first called by this name around 1887, although the phenomenon had been around for about 100 years before that. Its cause (overt damage to the brain, usually by an accident of some kind, but sometimes by brain disease) and effects (disruption in specific ways with characteristic error forms in spoken and written language—the dyslexia) are not in dispute. It is an aspect of dysphasia, which affects spoken as well as written forms of verbal

* What can/could be expected, assuming certain conditions.

11

;verbalcommunication—a condition which has been known about for about 200 years. A fundamental issue here is one that is central to the entire discussion on dyslexia and is that of distinguishing cause and effect. Dyslexia is *always* the effect—the resulting condition—of some cause. The causes and effects of these medical conditions are well documented. The causes of developmental dyslexia are manifold and the major ones will be described below.

The term 'dyslexia' means a dysfunction or disruption of the lexical or language-handling system of the brain. This system is composed of a number of structures in the brain, some of which apparently evolved quite late in the timescale of human development and others, like memory stores, which primarily serve other functions but are 'recruited' when necessary to support the processing of verbal language. These structures support functions in the brain, again some of which apparently evolved late in the day and others, like visual memory, that are 'recruited' to assist in the processing of language. These structures and functions are the province of study of medical doctors and psychologists, but some aspects are the subject of study by others, such as educators.

The term was first proposed in Germany by investigators researching the effects of brain damage or disease which included total or partial loss of a pre-existing ability to read and write.

Early investigators, medical doctors, including James Hinshelwood, a Glasgow eye surgeon, reported cases in which their patients exhibited difficulty in reading. Hinshelwood first reported the phenomenon in the UK in 1885. In 1896 Hinshelwood reported that reading by another of his patients ceased after a few words, at which point he apparently became 'blind' to words. The cause of this was subsequently shown to be temporary damage to parts of his brain.

For that reason, Hinshelwood used the term 'wordblindness' to describe the reading performance which was as if blind to words. This condition— **disruption of the ability to read as a result of damage**—was already called dyslexia by Kussmaul and Berlin and falls into the category of what is now called 'acquired' dyslexia.

The second, and by far the most common form of dyslexia, is relatively recent and is properly called developmental dyslexia because it is, in essence, the **failure—so far—to develop levels of fluency in reading and writing appropriate to what might be expected, given other abilities and opportunity to learn**—as distinct from disruption of a pre-existing ability to read and write.

This dysfunction, or disruption of the language-handling systems of the brain, therefore differs from the original form, in which **pre-existing** ability to read and write is disrupted whereas here, **appropriate levels of fluency** in the ability to read and write are **slower than expected in developing—or do not develop to the level of fluency expected**, which is itself a contentious issue.

It first emerged when, at around the same time as Hinshelwood's 'peculiar case of dyslexia', other medical doctors, WP Morgan in Sussex and J Kerr in Yorkshire, independently recorded cases of schoolboys having extraordinary difficulty in **developing** appropriate fluency in reading and writing; this was despite having at least average academic ability exhibited via the spoken form of the language, but who showed no evidence of damage or disease, other mental development being unaffected.

## Causation in developmental dyslexia

This form of dyslexia was also perceived as a medical condition whose cause was not obvious and therefore assumed to be a congenital, minimal and very localised form of brain damage or disease which prevented or obstructed the normal development of the ability to read and write.

It was not caused by lack of sufficient intellect nor by missing schooling, according to their tutors, although these possible causes—and indeed the concepts—do not appear to have ever been fully investigated by Morgan or Kerr. However, Hinshelwood later reviewed similar patients of his and showed that poor tuition **was** involved. He also showed and strongly contended that difficulties of this kind **could** and should be completely remedied by good and appropriate tuition.

Morgan, the physician responsible for providing medical services to the public school where the patient whose case he published was a pupil, recorded the precise nature of the performances of the individual concerned, but not the details of his educational history; this included all the complex factors in his learning process. It is possible that aspects of this deceptively simple process were the cause of the condition reported. However, it appears that in his cases, no attempt was made to investigate any educational or other cause of the specific learning difficulty.

These are central issues in any thorough investigation of cause and effect in relation to this phenomenon which need to be comprehensively addressed.

## Dyslexia and learning difficulty

Nevertheless, Morgan and Kerr, who reported similar cases in Yorkshire, maintained the proposition that brain damage was the cause of this difficulty in developing anticipated levels of fluency in reading and writing performances. But, because they could find no evidence of damage, they postulated the probability of minimal and very localised congenital damage or disease which was detectable only because of the unexpectedly poor reading performance. This is not dissimilar to Hinshelwood's actual conclusions and they may well have supposed that evidence of this damage would be found in a post-mortem examination (undertaken, if at all, long after they themselves had passed away, since the patients were much younger than they were).

In Morgan's report, published in the British Medical Journal, there is also the implied notion of use of other intellectual function—specifically academic attainment and later IQ—as a benchmark of expectation of the level of performance to which reading and writing ought to develop.

This notion later gained great popularity, becoming somewhat exaggerated and distorted by others in the process, taking it into the realms of education and learning theory and potentially away from medicine.

Successive writers have made much of the discrepancy between individuals' scholastic performances (which they assumed to be a valid benchmark of expectation of performance in reading and writing) and their reading and writing performances.

Since then, this issue of expectation—especially in the form of 'intelligence' expressed as 'IQ' or, rarely, other evidence of intellectual ability of the person concerned—has bedevilled investigation into the phenomenon of developmental dyslexia until fairly recently.

Much of the subsequent confusion and controversy may have been caused by this extrapolation and distortion of this notion by some 'thinkers' from different fields to cover very different concepts, many of which are educational rather than medical or even psychological.

The concept has, fortunately, been comprehensively demolished by careful research from about 1990 onwards—after which it has been increasingly and comprehensively shown to be invalid as a benchmark of expectation of performance in reading and writing, both of which are complex capabilities.

## Dyslexia and the notion of specific *learning* difficulty

The consequent further extrapolation of dyslexia as a difficulty in **learning**, which is specific to the development of fluency in the use of the written forms of the language, gave rise to the speculation that such difficulty was caused not by damage but instead by a maturational lag—a slowness to develop—or developmental failure in the brain structures and/or functions which subserve these abilities.

If these propositions of maturational lag and/or deficit are true, given the complexity of the structures, substructures and related structures which together make up the language-handling systems, then either all of these are similarly affected, or only some of them are, in the same way as the damage which causes loss of pre-existing fluency in the use of the language.

And since dyslexia affects only the written form of the language, that must mean only the structures and/or functions which are involved in the handling of the written language are affected. This, of course, includes the systems which handle sounds and awareness of phonology and visual and aural memory.

Now, if **all** the language handling systems are affected by a **general** deficit, one would expect the development—if there at all—to be 'normal' but retarded. The errors observed—the only overt indication of a problem—would be the same as those made by younger 'normal' learners. There are no recorded cases of **no** development taking place. The problems would therefore have to be either maturational delay in development of these systems or a **temporary** or **partial** deficit.

Additionally, a deficit in the systems might mean that the resultant dyslexia became permanent, especially after the age of eleven—although it is possible that it might be kick-started—whereas a delay caused by maturational **lag** would be temporary, with the development eventually coming to full function either by itself or by careful, appropriate stimulation via learning and practice.

In fact, all cases show some improvement over time, especially with careful supported learning. Alternatively, if only **some** subsystems were affected, the error forms exhibited should show characteristic error types as are seen in acquired dyslexia—and for the same reasons— except that the problem is not permanent damage but instead possibly temporary damage (the performance improves over time) or delay in maturation. Some researchers have shown apparent similarities between the error forms in developmental dyslexia and those in some types of acquired dyslexia.

However, these error forms are also typical of those made by normal readers—even skilled ones on occasion—and can be attributed to lack of or inappropriate application of strategies, skills and tactics when reading. In addition, it is possible that at least some of the errors produced by acquired dyslexics are a function of their attempts at learning to read all over again, perhaps from scratch.

It is well known that neural systems and pathways, including those in the brain, develop and increase in volume and strength in accordance with the use which is made of them. The more they are used in learning, development and the practice of specific functions, the more they will grow and the more effective and efficient they will be. Conversely, at a very early age and in extreme situations, some neural systems can atrophy, and perhaps even wither away.

One therefore has to be careful about attributing lack of development of neural systems and functions as the cause of poor reading development when this may actually be the consequence of it. Fortunately, with modern technology, it is possible to put this to the test by deliberate development of the abilities in question by appropriate means and observing the results over time on functional Magnetic resonance Imaging (fMRI) scans. Unfortunately these are very expensive and so not easily available.

And there is yet another major issue, not unrelated to the appropriateness of remedial tuition and learning. Given the complexity of the essential skills and knowledge to be learned—and the opportunity provided for them to be learned, as well as all the factors involved in learning *per se*—any failure in this learning, or in the provision of the opportunity to learn, must surely result in the same retarded or obstructed performances in reading and writing.

It is also well known that the provision of opportunity to learn—teaching—is very variable, with some schools and even some education authorities providing only a limited number of the essential skills and tactics for reading and writing for learning as a matter of policy. This is most evident in the fatuous 'phonics' versus 'whole books' or 'look and say' debate. The fact is, skilled as well as learner readers use a variety of strategies, tactics and skills to identify words and extract meaning from text. They therefore need to have **all** of the strategies, skills and tactics available at their fingertips for use when needed—if necessary on a trial and error basis. Failure to acquire one or more of these strategies, skills and tactics would therefore leave the reader partially disabled or at least disadvantaged. Some call this 'carefully nurtured dyslexia'! This situation is made much worse because of the vast difference between teaching and learning.

The opportunity to learn may well be properly presented to a class, but individual learners might not avail themselves of that opportunity for a variety of reasons. These can range from inattention caused by distraction, especially habitual distraction, or 'boredom'. The necessary motivation and commitment for learning to read are normally, for children at least, in the first instance not of their own making. It is somebody else's idea for them to learn to read and write.

The problem can become instead a struggle on the part of an individual to comprehend what is being taught—often because they have not come to the learning situation equipped with all the precursor skills, knowledge and understanding, the possession of which is an essential prerequisite for any hope of understanding this new information. One example of this might be a child who has entered school with very little experience of the precursor skills on which reading and writing are built, including communicating in the spoken form of the language. So, their ability to communicate, to receive and to give information, and their store of knowledge and information, might be inadequate for the subsequent building on of the ability to communicate in the written form of the language.

This struggle might, for some, be so destructive that it causes the learner to detach and perhaps withdraw from all learning, or become disruptive, or even become ill enough to miss significant amounts of schooling altogether. All too often such children are dismissed out of hand as incapable of learning—too dim to bother with—and so become the victims of carefully nurtured dyslexia.

The point is that if any of the essential building blocks of knowledge, skills and understanding are missed out for any of these 'normal' reasons, the net effect will be the same struggle to develop appropriate fluency in the use of the language—and this includes the underdevelopment of structure and function observable in fMRI scans, as is evident from other causes.

Given the variability in quality of educational provision as well as that involved in individual learning, these causes of developmental dyslexia are far more likely than any of the esoteric ones. With modern technology such as fMRI scanning now available, these propositions and related issues of cause and effect (eg. does learning to read cause the relevant brain structures and functions to develop) are testable and there is some evidence of this (Maguire, 2000).

It is also the case that until relatively recently, dyslexia—acquired dyslexia caused by brain damage—was said to be a subset of specific learning difficulty on the grounds of the reported incidence of each, being in the ratio of about 10:1. Putting aside the difficulty of accurate record-keeping in view of the many and often conflicting conceptions of each of these, given the British Psychological Society's Division of Educational and Child Psychology 1999 definition of developmental dyslexia and allowing the range of possible causes of this, it is more likely that specific learning difficulty is a subset of developmental dyslexia. Justification for this viewpoint is given below.

## Popular conceptions of what dyslexia is

Returning to the issue of the original conceptions of developmental dyslexia, it is unfortunate that these concepts have subsequently been modified by some to be a disease or physical developmental malfunction in its own right which **causes** other things, such as poor memory and other difficulties.

This has, in turn, led to a plethora of conceptions of cause and effect and of what dyslexia **is**. Some of these are no longer anything to do with medical conceptions and many 'definitions' or conceptions derived in this manner are mutually contradictory. Thus, there are now many conceptions or definitions of developmental dyslexia—some mutually exclusive, some soundly based on scientific research and some more on passionate belief, some downright weird, some not based on any proper evidence at all. Regrettably, for good remediation of the problem, the latter tend to be more popular with the general public than the former for a number of reasons, not always worthy ones.

The conceptions of what dyslexia 'is' most popularly held by the general public are, for example:

- 'sees some letters upside-down/backwards' (this is actually a visual/perceptual problem)

and/or

- 'hyperactive', and/or 'distractible' (this is caused by other things and can cause dyslexia)

and/or

- 'poor memory'—especially for sequences of information such as the days of the week or the months of the year or 'cannot remember a sequence of instructions'

and/or
- 'communicates well orally but written expression is poor'

and/or
- 'poor hand/eye co-ordination or clumsiness' (this may actually be dyspraxia)

and/or
- 'left-handedness' together with 'right-eye dominance'— or vice versa or any combination of one-side sensor and other side limb—allegedly indicating 'cross-laterality' (and of the involvement of the 'wrong' cerebral hemisphere dominating behaviour to the detriment of efficient language-handling—known generally as 'cerebral dominance'.

These are, in fact, somewhat inaccurate, popular descriptions of concomitants of poor reading or spelling. That is, **some of them** are **sometimes** also exhibited by those with poor reading or spelling and may be the cause, but by no means all are evident, or even any of them in all cases. Moreover, if they do appear, this is only coincidentally, or along with, the poor reading or spelling and are likely to be caused by other things and that, too, can be relatively easily ascertained. They are neither characteristics nor 'symptoms' of developmental dyslexia. If they were, the non-appearance of some, if not all of them, in many, if not most, currently diagnosed developmental dyslexics would logically have to mean that such persons are not really dyslexic.

Unfortunately, 'developmental dyslexia' is differentiated by the adherents of this conception from 'ordinary' poor readers or spellers on the grounds that these are 'symptoms' of a mysterious ailment called 'dyslexia', and although this is presented as a scientific, or at least technical, conclusion, it may actually be largely political!

## Developmental dyslexia educationally defined

In 1999, after years of considering the evidence, a review body of the BPsS DECP (1999) concluded that:

> *'Developmental dyslexia is evident when accurate and fluent word reading and/or spelling develops very incompletely or with great difficulty despite appropriate learning opportunities—that is, learning opportunities which are effective for the great majority of children.'*

BPsS DECP (1999)

This concept of **developmental** dyslexia—the failure, so far, to develop levels of fluency in reading and writing appropriate to what might be expected, given other abilities and opportunity to learn—can arguably have a number of possible causes. These, including the evidence from the latest research, will be given in detail later.

## Other conceptions of developmental dyslexia

Over the last 110 years, dyslexia has been said to be caused by (and later distorted by some to actually be) a range of things including those listed below in some detail. They are listed in the order in which they have appeared following the original phenomenon of (acquired) dyslexia and most continue to, at least, implicitly accept dyslexia as the condition of inordinate difficulty in developing appropriate levels of fluency in the ability to read and write, and differ only in the supposed cause. In other words, the medical model is broadly retained, although, in a few cases, at some point comprehensively distorted.

Where appropriate, the approximate date of emergence of each version of the concept—which differs for the most part in suggested cause—is given, along with the person, doctor of medicine or psychologist responsible for the conception.

Since first recorded by Hinshelwood, then Kerr and Morgan, what is now called developmental dyslexia has been variously postulated to be: a difficulty in (learning to) read and write, caused by:

**a) A congenital defect**—NOT inadequate conventional instruction or inadequate IQ:

The possibility of a congenital defect was first postulated by Hinshelwood and later more directly referred to in his book published in 1917, and at least implied by Morgan (Pringle) and Kerr in 1896. This was also the conclusion of the 1968 symposium of the World Federation of Neurology (WFN) which retained the same basic ideas of cause and effect as the medical model of acquired dyslexia—the effect being dyslexia similar in conception to that of acquired dyslexia. The WFN definition excluded those who did not experience normal education and those with 'inadequate IQ' from being judged to be dyslexic. These views have since been strongly challenged on a number of grounds—not least being, 'what is adequate IQ' and what is 'conventional instruction'?

One British member of the World Federation of Neurology is said to have concluded that the cause of the dyslexia was a selective deterioration of the myelin sheathing (which enhances the conveyance of the electrical impulse along nerves) of the nerves in the brain—as is seen in multiple sclerosis. However, it has never been explained why this should attack only the language-handling parts of the brain and why no characteristic errors, such as are seen in acquired, brain damage dyslexia, appear. The errors formed in developmental dyslexia are generally indistinguishable from those made 'normally'. The same is true of the suggested effects of products such as gluten and fatty acids.

At the same time, the notion first implied by Morgan and Kerr, also related to the exclusion of inadequate schooling and inadequate IQs—that dyslexia could only be experienced by those with higher than average IQs—the notion of 'specific learning difficulty', became very popular, not always for the best of reasons. The others were presumably just too 'thick' to learn. In view of the complexity of what has to be learned, as well as the complexity of learning *per se*, substantial argument can be made against this.

This 'diagnosis' of developmental dyslexia indicated by an unexpectedly poor performance in the context of the proposition that reading performance should match 'IQ', as measured by tests such as the Weschler Intelligence Scale for Children (WISC) and the Weschler Adult Intelligence Scale (WAIS)—based on correlation between the two—became almost standard practice for many. The basis of this has also been seriously questioned.

**b) 'A hereditary' and/or 'genetic defect'** (first suggested by Hinshelwood around 1907):
Moving on from his view of the cause of the struggle to develop the ability to use one or more aspects of the written form of the language, Hinshelwood suggested that cases of familial incidence brought to his notice might suggest genetic inheritance. He appeared to suggest, however, quite logically, that the inheritance is (possibly) of a defective neural structure which is specific to the aspect of the language handling system, particularly that of visual memory. This appears to have been subsequently distorted to the notion that **dyslexia**—the consequence of such inadequate structural or functional inheritance—is itself what is inherited. This distortion, whether of misunderstanding or a deliberate act, may well be the origin of the absurd notion that **dyslexia** is some kind of inherited brain disorder and not, as it actually is, the **consequence** of that.

At some time during this period, the notion emerged that developmental dyslexia was an educational and not a medical issue and, in 1981, the British Medical Association publicly expressed this view. However, this depends on what is perceived to be the cause and, based on Hinshelwood's views, if the cause is deficit—or even maturational lag—in the language-handling neural pathways which inhibits development of reading skills, and not the other way round, it may still be the province of neurologists, even though they can do little about it.

The BMA's comment may have been a reaction to the emergence of the now popular conception, noted above, of dyslexia as a mysterious ailment which causes or has 'symptoms' which include memory problems and/or a different way of thinking, as well as a host of other things. The evidence to support this conception is not hard to find and has, in some aspects, been comprehensively disproved—but it is, nevertheless, popular with the general population—again not always for the best of reasons.

c) **Inadequate/erratic scanning** (e.g. Pavlidis, c1981):
Pavlidis suggested a diagnostic system for detection of developmental dyslexia which consisted of excluding possible causes, such as those also excluded by the WFN in 1968, and extended this list considerably. This is known as a 'wastebasket' procedure in that, when all disallowed is discarded, dyslexia is what is left.

Pavlidis also concluded from his studies that the cause of this dyslexia was the unsystematic saccadic eye movements exhibited by the sufferers. This could explain phenomena such as letter and word 'reversals'. Unfortunately for this theory, it was realised these individuals' unsystematic eye movements when reading were **a consequence of their not yet having learned how to read in a skilled way** and when they did, their unsystematic eye movements disappeared. This phenomenon can be invoked in skilled readers.

d) **Scotopic sensitivity syndrome** (Irlen, c1980; Stein, c1980/ 2003; Wilkins, c1980):
This is the phenomenon of text appearing to 'jump', thus making reading, especially for learners, difficult. This is of course a **visual** problem, as is the later suggestion that the cause of dyslexia is, instead, a very slightly unco-ordinated passage of signals from the eyes to the part of the brain where vision is first processed—the occipital lobe at the back of the head. There are two separate neural pathways—the magnocellular and the parvocellular—along which the pulses normally pass and, if the signals passing along these from the eyes are not synchronous, the resultant vision will be blurred because the same information is received in the occipital lobe from each pathway milliseconds apart. This is the province of optometrists and for them to remedy.

Persons who do not normally experience it can be relatively easily made to experience jumping of text by presenting them with very closely spaced lines of small text, or even just thick black lines with small white space between them. The apparent jumping (a visual illusion) can be made to stop by spacing the lines further apart. It can also be stopped by filtering the light absorbed by the eyes when looking at the text or lines with coloured spectacles. About £200 was charged for some of these spectacles, but the same affect can be achieved with coloured acetate overlays costing about ten pence. Different people who normally experience text 'jumping' report one colour of acetate or another solves the problem for them. Which colour works for them seems to be a matter of personal preference but Stein has recently shown that the most effective hue is blue.

e) **Cross-laterality reversed perception of visual images** (Orton, c1937):
There are several 'theories' about cause in this particular vein.

Among the very good work done by the American medical doctor, Samuel Orton, is his suggestion—which since then has been used by some to justify the phenomenon of letter and word 'reversals'—that what the left eye sees is passed to the right hemisphere of the brain and what the right eye sees is passed to the left hemisphere, the area which is known to be the primary processing centre of verbal language (neither oral nor written but in electro-chemical impulse form at this point).

This conflicts with what was known even then about how the visual system in the brain actually works— expanded later as a result of experiments in the 1940s and 1950s and comprehensively shown to be wrong. However, that has not deterred some current proponents.

f) **Left-handedness**:
This is a particular version of the cross-laterality theory which has also been shown to be quite wrong. Having to write from left to right across the page clearly presents practical difficulties for left-handers in languages which are written this way, but not for those whose languages are written right to left, like Hebrew—and bottom to top **and** right to left, like Chinese.

Research has also shown that the proportion of those experiencing reading difficulties in the left-handed population is no greater than that in the right-handed majority.

g) **Unusual brain structure**:
(*see also 'What do you mean 'developmental'? below)

- Of the temporal planum (a flattish surface on the underside of each temporal [middle] lobe of the cerebra)—good readers have enlarged left temporal planum, 'dyslexics' (uncertain how defined) have symmetric plana or sometimes a slightly enlarged right temporal planum (e.g. Geschwind, 1976).

*Less developed neural subsystems which carry the functions of reading and writing*

- (See Maguire *et al*, 2000), as well as current studies of the same phenomenon at the Institute of Neurology.

**h) Unusual brain function:**
(\*see 'What do you mean 'developmental'? below)

- Poorer readers, ?dyslexics have less activity in the left hemisphere during reading related tasks (fMRI scans) (reported by Snowling).

For further information about the involvement of brain structure and function on learning to read, see page 78

**i) A 'syndrome' which starts with (undefined) 'less developed' cognitive function** (Snowling, 2000, citing Vellutino, 1997) resulting in poorer letter knowledge and number naming skills but **no** difference in IQ in a sample of American children of kindergarten age. This also results in poorer verbal short-term memory, phonological awareness and speed of naming in a sample of American children in first grade in school; i.e. poorer precursor skills/basis for learning to read!—which is what actually differentiates those resistant to intervention from those not so resistant to intervention, according to Vellutino.
NB: these are present both in generally poor readers **and** those with 'specific learning difficulties'. Poorer precursor skills can also emanate from inadequate pre-school development, most probably caused by socio-cultural factors.

**j) A 'syndrome' of causation** in which early spoken form speech and language difficulties cause inadequate phonological representation in the relevant language-handling structures of the brain—which, in turn, results in inadequate phonological awareness and therefore inadequate skills in application of this—which results in inadequate development of appropriate levels of fluency of skills of reading and writing.

For a more detailed consideration of these two syndromes, see page 80.

*Alternatively*, it is....

k)   A 'maturational lag'or deficit claimed by some to affect parts of the brain not always known to be part of the language-handling neurological systems, such as the cerebellum and vestibular systems. Moreover, the more extreme versions of these propositions insist that the sufferer is otherwise very intelligent and even gifted in other ways.

The cerebellum is, however, part of the autonomic arousal system—the brain system which controls alertness and therefore optimum efficiency/effectiveness in responding to a stimulus, or in readiness to learn—and it is known that this can be a major factor in learning in general and potentially, therefore, specifically in learning to read and write. This can happen if the learner is understimulated, at the lower end of the arousal curve—or 'dozy'—or if they are overstimulated, over the top of the arousal curve—OTT or hyperactive. This latter condition may explain why drugs such as Ritalin—an amphetamine stimulant—can have beneficial effects for some learners, although it is more of a puzzle when it helps the overstimulated. What it **may** be doing is helping the neural pathways to operate more efficiently instead of spraying information all over the place at random. Further research on that is needed. It is also suggested that poor development of the vestibular system can cause visual difficulties—rather like dyspraxia can have visual difficulties as a concomitant—and in either case, such visual difficulties may be the cause of dyslexia.

There are other 'global' suggested causes, such as inadequacy of fatty acids and negative reactions to gluten or wheat-laden products, which are thought by some to have deleterious effects on learning to read. There is, though, a question on why such effects should be selective, as some claim.

*Alternatively again*, it is...

l)    **The end of a chain of inference for those in one of the major sub-groups** (Specific Learning Difficulty ('SPLD')) which goes something like...:

The affected person's performance in reading and/or spelling is significantly lower than their 'IQ'. Their 'IQ' is at least average (usually higher) and it's only their reading/spelling which is affected. That must mean something is obstructing that development alone. That something must be dyslexia!—which **causes—or a manifestation of which is**—difficulty in reading or spelling!
    The following might or might not be related...

- A different way of processing information/thinking caused by:

    - unusual formations in the language handling systems of the brain

    - abnormalities in the cerebellum.

- A 'different' brain structure and/or function which manifests itself in several ways, such as high IQ, poor reading/spelling, excellent spatial abilities, poor memory/ forgetfulness, disorganised thinking and behaviour.

    It is alleged by the adherents of this conception of dyslexia that dyslexics have a different way of thinking from the rest of us. Some go even further and assert that dyslexics have extraordinarily well-developed spatial abilities, such as might be useful for architects or graphic artists. In fact there is no evidence of this. The incidence of those with better than average spatial abilities is no greater in dyslexics than it is in the rest of the population. For those who are better than average, it is more likely that this has come about as a result of compensating for difficulty in developing adequate levels of fluency in the use of the written language and finding alternative ways of acquiring information and expressing themselves.

Extreme conceptions such as this appear to have evolved through misunderstanding and/or distortion of the original concepts—at times and for some adherents, becoming completely detached from these while retaining traces of their scientific respectability.

## Dyslexia is a complex issue

Dyslexia—both forms—has at least five aspects: scientific, technical, social, emotional and political (including practical, educational policy and access to funds).

In this book, it will be argued that the only tenable definition of developmental dyslexia is that of the BPsS DECP (1999), which is very similar to that of the original (acquired) dyslexia. It will also be argued that there is a range of possible causes of this condition, including 'normal' failures of education provision. Argument will also be made for the propositions that: 1) developmental dyslexia as defined by the BPsS DECP can be caused by a range of things—often two or more causes acting in concert; 2) this condition is not limited to those whose general intellect is well above their reading ability; and 3) this condition can be minimised if not eradicated by careful, thorough investigation of cause(s) and application of an appropriate remedial action—**provided that the learner has sufficient motivation and commitment to such learning.**

Detailed consideration of those will follow the introduction of the practical value of being able to read and communicate in the written form of the language and a brief description of what these faculties actually are. This is necessary to make this deceptively simple, but actually complex, phenomenon easier to understand.

## So what can we accept as developmental dyslexia—the distinguishing features?

Both forms can be caused by damage to very specific areas—visual memory storage areas and/or connecting neural pathways.

Acquired dyslexia is loss of pre-existing ability. Developmental dyslexia is failure to develop that ability—but **not** completely, only to **the level of fluency anticipated**. That, of course, raises many questions, not least about on what basis is the expectation founded and why? What is the justification for that?

Developmental dyslexia can be caused by a large range of things other than damage. A large proportion of these may be normal causes. The probability of normal causation is much greater than any other possible cause.

It **might** also be the consequence of neural maturational lag (or it may cause that). This is not true of acquired dyslexia. However, the maturational lag might be the **consequence** of failure, so far, to develop appropriate levels of the ability to read. This is a testable hypothesis which can be tested using modern technology (e.g. fMRI scanning).

It **might** be caused by a deficit. However, this deficit—a piece of the system missing, itself a failure to develop—would result in permanent failure of the ability to use the written form of the language to develop, and probably result in no development rather than retarded development. There are no such cases recorded except in cases of overt developmental failure which is usually more global.

### Distinguishing the developmental dyslexic from other poor readers

Poor readers who are specifically reading retarded (the SRR group) and those who are generally retarded (the GRR group) all struggle to develop fluency in the ability to use the written form of the language. In the former, this is not anticipated; in the latter, because they are perceived as generally intellectually inferior, rightly or wrongly, it is.

This is often used as a distinguishing feature but in practice the factor most commonly used to distinguish specifically retarded readers from generally backward readers is IQ—variously conceived.

As a consequence of this, however, an essential difference between dyslexics and other poor readers means that, for the former, difficulty in development of the faculties of reading and communicating in the written form of the language is, or should be, relatively easily overcome.

Recent research on dyslexics, identified as those exhibiting 'significant discrepancy' between their IQ and performances in use of the written form of the language, did not find that such discrepancy-defined 'dyslexics' had an especially poor prognosis. Instead, there was some evidence that SRR did better than GRR—contradicting the idea that they cannot learn—and the differences in progress made by these groups not only varied over time but sometimes one and sometimes the other made better progress.

Ultimately, the only consistent difference between the two groups was the difference in IQ. This also contradicts any suggestion that 'dyslexics' somehow have different brain arrangements or functioning, or think differently from the rest of us—or indeed that those exhibiting specific reading difficulties are the only group suffering from dyslexia.

Moreover, other noted authorities in this field have shown that the correlation between IQ and reading is—for what it's worth—at best only 0.3. That is, only about 9 per cent of the variance is shared and there is no implication of causation of one by the other in either direction. Most respected researchers interpret this as the final, conclusive evidence that there is no validity in the 'discrepancy' model for identifying or 'diagnosing' dyslexia. In other words, as research by the BPsS DECP has also concluded, 'IQ' has little or nothing to do with dyslexia. In addition, also contrary to popular mythology based on a supposed list of 'symptoms' or 'indicators' of dyslexia, research has shown a different picture.

Generally poor readers (the GRR group) showed more neurological 'soft' signs such as movement disorders and clumsiness—said by some to be symptoms of the mysterious brain disease called dyslexia found only in 'intelligent' people. They also showed more neurological impairments such as epilepsy than the specific reading retarded (SRR) group—which may be inferred as a lack of indication of inadequate brain development. In addition, the SRR group were better at the 'finger agnosia' test (a test often used as a 'sign' or 'symptom' of dyslexia), at sentence memory and at object naming—all also said by some to be indicators of a mysterious brain disease called dyslexia.

Both groups show raised incidence of indicators of late onset of speech, of speech and language problems and of incidence of this in the family. The groups did, however, differ in respect of SRR having more complex language use—which is consistent with their higher 'IQ'.

The BPsS DECP definition of developmental dyslexia is a descriptive term for extraordinary difficulty in developing appropriate levels of fluency in the skills of reading and writing and/or an incomplete development of these. It is a description of the observed situation—the production of errors and extraordinary difficulty in improving performance.

Recent research has identified among poor readers who are otherwise indistinguishable, a sub-group whose defining characteristic is a relatively poor (least good) response to intervention. If this is a sustainable finding then **this** may be the distinguishing characteristic or cause of specific reading retardation. There can, however, be 'normal' reasons for that, such as poor development of precursor skills and knowledge. One eminent authority on the subject already suggests that those particularly resistant to improvement given remedial tuition might be the 'true dyslexics'. On the other hand, the same authority also cites research which indicates that 'true dyslexics' differ from other poor readers on 'cognitive profile'. In practice, the dimensions of this which are cited—poor phonological awareness and related phonological skills, verbal short-term memory, and slowness in rapid naming—are all what those such as Goswami call precursor skills—and these have already been identified as the likely cause of resistance to intervention.

Precursor skills are the abilities which children bring to school with them on first entry and the variability across individuals is enormous. They are also abilities which can be developed in pre-school years, influenced by their 'environment', which includes social, cultural and other aspects as well as the physical environment.

In summary then, current research is indicating that the 'true' dyslexics are those who are more resistant to remedial tuition than others with the same difficulties and, significantly, also that this resistance may be laid at the door of inadequate development of the precursor skills for reading and writing, including poor social and communication skills and especially language skills in those with early speech or hearing problems.

Poor development of these precursor skills and speech development are, therefore, potential causes of developmental dyslexia, or at least potentially predispose those unfortunate enough to suffer them to later development of developmental dyslexia as described by the BPsS DECP. Addressing these at the appropriate time could well mean avoiding developmental dyslexia altogether. That being so, there are significant implications for the activities of health visitors and nursery teachers and nurses for the pre-schoolers.

## Developmental dyslexic or just a poor reader?

The label 'dyslexic' is said by some to be not applicable when the cause of the problems is, for example inadequate 'IQ' or schooling or obvious visual or hearing difficulties—but it may be quite wrong to deny that those for whom these are the cause are also dyslexic as defined by the BPsS DECP in 1999. It may be wrong because these difficulties produce exactly the same effect described.

It is also said by some that the term is applicable only when the struggle to develop appropriate levels of fluency is seen in those who have developed their other intellectual abilities 'normally'. In such cases the problem is also called specific learning difficulty. That's because inadequate development of appropriate levels of fluency in the use of the written language may be the *only* difficulty they have.

However, limiting the label of dyslexic to this group alone is also questionable. This is because, as recent research also shows, the nature of their difficulties and their cause is no different from the difficulties experienced by those whose other intellectual development so far is also restricted. Unfortunately, this group is usually but wrongly perceived to be intellectually unable to do any better than they do.

The reality is that, given access to information in the written form enhances intellectual development. The restricted general intellectual development of this group may therefore be a consequence of their restricted fluency in the use of the written language. In other words, the difference between them and those whose restriction is only in use of the written language is that the latter have founds ways of circumventing the problem and acquiring information by other means and the others haven't yet been helped to do that. This is quite easy to demonstrate.

## What *does* cause developmental dyslexia?

As may be seen from the conceptions above, the majority of experts agree—and have agreed since its inception—that developmental dyslexia is the description of a condition in which someone learning to use the written form of the language exhibits a poorer-than-expected level of fluency in this, as well as an inordinate struggle to improve their performance. The concept has long been disputed but most of the dispute is, and has been, about how this condition comes about.

Since the condition was first mooted around 1896, the cause has been followed up many blind alleys, one after another. Fortunately, as our understanding of how the brain works has improved by leaps and bounds, our understanding of why appropriate anticipated levels of fluency in use of the written language by some learners has also markedly improved.

### Possible causes of developmental dyslexia

It bears repeating that developmental dyslexia can be caused by a large range of things other than damage. A large proportion of these things may be normal causes. The probability of normal causation is much greater than any other possible cause.

It *might* also be the consequence of neural maturational lag (or it may cause that). This is not true of acquired dyslexia.

However, the maturational lag might be the *consequence* of failure—so far—to develop appropriate levels of ability to read. This is a testable hypothesis which can be tested using modern technology (i.e. fMRI scanning).

It *might* be caused by a deficit. However, this deficit—a piece of the system missing—itself a failure to develop, would result in permanent failure of the ability to use the written form of the language to develop—and probably result in no development rather than retarded development. There are no such cases recorded except in cases of overt developmental failure which is usually more global.

The range of cause(s) of persistent, almost intractable difficulty in developing appropriate levels of fluency in reading and writing, the condition described by the BPsS DECP as developmental dyslexia, embraces a range of 'normal' ones, including not being taught or not learning for a range of reasons. These alone can cause non- or under-development of the critical factors involved in learning and performance in general as well as those specifically necessary for learning to read and write, all of which may interact with each other, making the situation complex.

In an interesting paper presented recently to the annual conference of the British Psychological Society (Goswami, 2002), Usha Goswami, a respected researcher in this field, suggested that a large part of the problem is the complexity and difficulty of learning the English language itself. This is supported by research into reading difficulties in other languages worldwide—all of which have a much more regular sound to graphic (letter) correspondence than English does.

However, in the view of some recent researchers, the condition is caused by a difficulty in forming phonological representation in the brain's language-handling systems, which may ultimately be the consequence of poorly developed precursor skills and knowledge for reading and writing. This is said to give rise to inadequate development of phonological awareness of these structures and therefore the skills/abilities in using these and, in turn, word identification skills.

Other research suggests that the cause of this inadequate phonological representation of the sound structures of the spoken language in the language-handling systems of the brain is deficits/inadequacies in early spoken language development. It should be noted that this affects both 'ordinary' poor readers (the 'generally backward') and those whose reading difficulty is said to be specific (on the grounds of 'IQ' scores which are higher than reading/spelling scores).

However, there seems to be little research into the effects of deliberate remedial 'teaching' of these, or into what in the way of relevant development children bring with them when they start school—and why.

There are many 'normal' reasons for/causes of the condition described by the BPsS DECP, but these are largely ignored—possibly because learning to read seems to be so easy and quick. Use of the written form of the language for communicating in writing and for reading that communication is a learned skill, as is the use of the spoken form.

Almost everybody is obliged to participate in using spoken language to make their wishes known and to get what they want from a very early age. Learning is informal and intensive. Use of the written form of the language is not quite like that.

In most societies, learning to read and write—essential skills for further learning and development—starts off as somebody else's idea (teacher's, parents') and is usually very formal and rigidly structured—and not necessarily related to actual life requirements at that point in their little lives. It's possible, at least initially, to get by without them. Of course there are notable individual exceptions to this.

The process is deceptively simple, evolving as it does over a period of years and usually based on reasonably successful use of the spoken language, which thereafter develops alongside it in relation to perceived demands.

Poor reading and writing (properly communicating in the written form of the language to distinguish it from the physical act of handwriting)—including developmental dyslexia—relative to expectations of performance of these, of whatever kind, are therefore a failure to learn these skills. This may be apparently specific to use of the written language or set in a context of other equally poor intellectual skills or knowledge development (anyone ever heard of dys-geography?) but, given the actual complexity of development of the skills of reading and writing (see the next page for a summary), this is not surprising. There are a great many places where it can go wrong—for 'normal' reasons.

Nor does it stop there. It's often said that evidence of 'normal schooling' means that the poor reading**/developmental dyslexia must be caused by something else.

This can be challenged because, as we all know, teaching is not the same as learning. Most of us have been in a situation where 'good' teaching has been taking place but learning hasn't—at least not for everybody present. That's because of all of the factors involved in learning which are **additional** to those needed to successfully develop appropriate levels of the skills of using the written language.

** Used here to mean all aspects of the use of the written form of the language

## Stepwise development of the skills of reading and communicating in writing: SUMMARY

```
┌─────────────────┐        ┌──────────────────────┐
│     Reading     │        │    Communicating     │
│                 │        │      in writing      │
│                 │        │       Spelling       │
└─────────────────┘        └──────────────────────┘
```

**Underpinning and enabling LANGUAGE skills**
**e.g. segmentation and blending**

**Underpinning or enabling NON-LANGUAGE skills**
**e.g. memory and perception**

**Physical and physiological skills**
**e.g. visual acuity motor skills**

**Controllable motivation and commitment to learn**
**to read and communicate in writing**

The process starts at the bottom—although which of the first three steps comes first is debatable—and ends, insofar as it ever does, in appropriate levels of skill.

This is a summary. Something like the full set of actual skills and knowledge needed is on the next page.

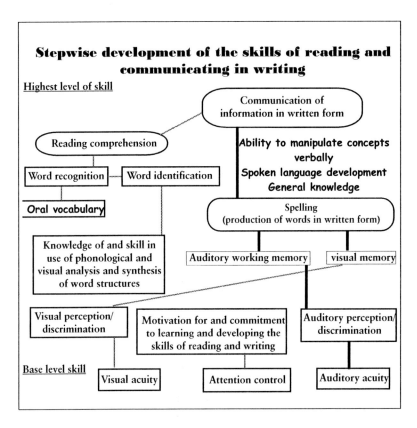

**Stepwise development of the skills of reading and communicating in writing**

Highest level of skill

Communication of information in written form

Reading comprehension

Word recognition — Word identification

Ability to manipulate concepts verbally
Spoken language development
General knowledge

Oral vocabulary

Spelling (production of words in written form)

Knowledge of and skill in use of phonological and visual analysis and synthesis of word structures

Auditory working memory    visual memory

Visual perception/ discrimination

Motivation for and commitment to learning and developing the skills of reading and writing

Auditory perception/ discrimination

Base level skill

Visual acuity    Attention control    Auditory acuity

Here again the process starts at the bottom.

The highlighted notes are pieces of information obtained from such as the WISC/WAIS which can be used to evaluate the information obtained from reading and spelling tests. Other tests can be used diagnostically to produce information about adequacy of skills development for the ultimate purpose.

It may be seen from these diagrams that there are many places where failure to learn or have the opportunity to learn— i.e. be taught—can have disastrous effects on the further development of the ultimate ability to communicate in the written form of the language and/or to read that communication. Missing pieces may also cause resistance to learning to otherwise successful remedial tuition.

The factors involved in learning *per se* are on the next page.

## Factors in learning *per se*

These include:

- motivation, attention and commitment—a genuine wish to learn **these** skills and associated knowledge
- a knowledge base appropriate and sufficient for further development of the requisite skills and knowledge—necessary to make sense of what's being taught (i.e. learning)
- an appropriately organised store in which to sort, classify, relate, manipulate (consider) and retrieve the incoming information
- information presented to the learner in such as way that it makes sense **to them personally.**

This may require learning facilitation as opposed to teaching by the teacher and it may be quite difficult for any teacher to determine the nature of the 'ground for learning'/readiness to learn for any given individual—especially in a class of 30 six-year-olds.

**And some of the other factors necessary as an adequate basis for learning to read:**

- Scanning skills and techniques; blending techniques
- Habitual arousal state (from 'dozy' to 'hyperactive'/over-the-top [of the arousal curve?])
- Adequate concept formation/intellectual development (especially for development beyond the 'mechanical')
- Adequate oral language handling development
- Capacity to use and adapt extended forms of spoken language
- Sociability/habitual tendency to interact and communicate
- Adequate vocabulary ('verbally-mediated concept store').

Therefore, successful remediation must follow and be informed by thorough investigation, involving trial and error investigative tuition and, where appropriate, all of the possible reasons for, or factors involved in, the observed poor performance.

## More possible causes

The condition described by the BPsS DECP as developmental dyslexia can also be caused by a range of other things, some of which may not be obvious until uncovered by thorough investigation. These include fine levels of visual or hearing inadequacies which are not detected by the usual gross sight or hearing tests but are such that they will restrict, if not obstruct, development of appropriate levels of fluency in reading and writing.

Other possible causes, when present, **are** obvious. A moment's thought will bolster the realisation that the things asserted by some to be 'symptoms' of the 'mystery ailment', said by them to be dyslexia, are actually things which will **cause** dyslexia as defined by the BPsS DECP. For example, people who are habitually disorganised in their thinking and behaviour will find it difficult to learn complex and demanding skills and strategies, such as phonological awareness and application of that knowledge, precisely **because** their habitual manner of thinking is disorganised. The same is true of those who have overt memory, visual or hearing problems.

In summary, developmental dyslexia as defined by the BPsS DECP may also be attributable to:

- Visual difficulties (especially the hard-to-detect ones, such as convergence, ciliary motor control difficulties, unestablished reference eye)
- Visuo-spatial perception difficulties
- Motor control difficulties
- Hearing difficulties (especially the not-normally-tested- for ones, such as phoneme discrimination, as well as all the abilities related to awareness of the phonological structure of the spoken language and the ability to apply the related skills and tactics fluently)
- Memory difficulties (those related to the acts of writing and reading)

- Organisational difficulties (disorganised physical and/or mental behaviour)
- Inadequate development of precursor and enabling skills, such as phonological analysis
- Inadequate oral vocabulary and fluency in use of the spoken language.

In developmental dyslexia, the errors made are no different from those made by others, especially by other poor readers. These errors and the inadequate development of fluency can also be explained by inadequacy in (development of) one or more of the skills which underpin reading and writing.

The only way to unequivocally ascertain cause is to progressively identify and eliminate all possible 'normal' causes. During this process, perhaps using the list of possible causes, observations of performance and other procedures and devices, the cause or causes will become evident. If anything inexplicable is left at the end of that process, it may be a mysterious cause—but the dyslexia is still the result of that cause.

## Identifying developmental dyslexia in the classroom

### The phenomenon of developmental dyslexia defined educationally

> *'Developmental dyslexia is evident when accurate and fluent word reading and/or spelling develops very incompletely or with great difficulty despite appropriate learning opportunities—that is, learning opportunities which are effective for the great majority of children.'*
>
> British Psychological Society (1999)

That is to say, dyslexia is a descriptive term for extraordinary or unexpected difficulty in developing appropriate levels of fluency in the skills of reading and writing and/or an incomplete development of these.

Not all poor performances in reading and communicating in the written language—which includes spelling—can be called developmental dyslexia. The definition of developmental dyslexia is given elsewhere. In essence, this is poor performances in the use of the written language which are more resistant than usual to intervention (remedial tuition). Poor performances in using the written language—including those described as dyslexia—can be caused by a range of things. These, too, are listed elsewhere.

For the reasons listed elsewhere, all poor performances in using the written language should be put right as soon as possible. This can be achieved by appropriate tuition and, in the case of developmental dyslexia, this may only be a little different from that required by any other form of poor use of the written language.

In order to produce the most appropriate learning programme, it is necessary to identify as precisely as possible what one is dealing with. It therefore helps to be able to identify developmental dyslexia and its cause(s) and this may be achieved by the following process.

**What would you see?**

- Poor performance in reading (word identification) and spelling which was: a) significantly worse than class peers (who have the same educational experience); b) poorer than was expected from this individual. (What constitutes legitimate expectation in this context is a large issue in its own right.) In adults, it might be less obvious

- A failure to comprehend the concepts and/or acquire/develop the constituent/enabling knowledge and skills, for example phonics.

At this point further investigation should be triggered.

## What would lead you to suspect dyslexia (BPsS DECP definition)?

- Little or no improvement in response to tuition which was appropriate to learning to read—**provided that** the learner was clearly trying to learn.

At this point developmental dyslexia might be suspected and further investigation of possible cause(s), then more personalised remedial tuition, should be implemented.

Note: Developmental dyslexia is a sub-class of poor reading performance. 'Specific learning difficulty' is a sub-class of developmental dyslexia. The **causes** of reading difficulties—including developmental dyslexia—are manifold and listed elsewhere.

## When would this be evident?

Given that learning to read is taking place from school entry to about age seven, performance discrepancy might not be evident until then. However, a struggle to learn or keep pace might be evident from the outset.

If screening for the precursor skills, e.g. adequate spoken form usage (pre-school) and letter knowledge, sight word learning and number skills (naming), is undertaken on entry or shortly thereafter, absence of these might alert the teacher to the likelihood of struggle to learn to write and read. Parents may be able to provide information on these if made aware of what to look for. If unaddressed these might evolve into poorer than average verbal short-term memory, phonological awareness and speed of naming.

In adults, the problem may be obscured—not least because of compounding social and emotional factors—but the fundamental phenomenon is the same. For the same reasons, resistance to remediation may be more entrenched.

## What residual evidence should there be of this?

- Records of tuition provided for class
- Records of specific remedial tuition provided for an individual showing signs of falling behind.

## What can be done about it

Contrary to the opinion of those who claim that dyslexia is for life and nothing much can be done to even relieve the situation, there is substantial evidence to show that not only can the situation be improved, but the problem(s) can be eliminated and the performances brought up to normal levels.

Even Hinshelwood, whose scientific investigations led to the recognition of several aspects of both acquired and developmental dyslexia, reported from working with his patient that a) most of his cases of developmental dyslexia had clear evidence of inadequate tuition; and b) given appropriate tuition—and he had a bit to say about what that was which will strike a chord in modern educational circles—and perseverance, especially the latter, the developmental dyslexia patients and even some of the damage dyslexia patients' performance could be brought up to normal standards. More recent organisations such as the Dyslexia Institute have had similar results from their teaching.

The trick is to find out exactly what's causing the problem then institute a personalised learning programme which will remedy the situation. Early detection is important. The sooner such problems are discovered and appropriate help given, the sooner they will be alleviated or overcome.

It is then imperative that the all of the possible causes of the problem—obvious and not so obvious—are identified (by the appropriate specialist professionals, such as optometrists, where necessary) and minimised, if not removed. Whether preventative, or as a response to need made evident by assessment, dealing with the situation will require a thorough exposition and listing of all the possible causes of the observed situation, recognising that this may be the interaction of a number of factors and therefore complex. This in turn makes a thorough investigation of problems and causes even more necessary, followed by provision of a learning programme derived from this information.

This learning programme also has certain other essential characteristics which make it, too, complex and so requires a suitably skilled learning facilitator or tutor to manage it. It has to be personalised—tailored to the individual for whom it has been designed, focused, in that it addresses each of the difficulties or causes that have been identified in the assessment which led to its production, intensive and flexible—adapted as the learner' s skills and needs change in response to the programme.

In addition to all that, the learning programme should not be delivered in isolation. Reading and writing are essential skills for everything we do. It is therefore necessary to practise and consolidate the advances in skills, knowledge and techniques, made as a result of the success of the learning programme, in normal settings such as the classroom or work or other normal application in which they are used.

## Options upon detection

Once developmental dyslexia has been identified there are three possible responses:

- The condition can be remediated by removal of the cause(s), followed by intensive specialist tuition to bring performance up to appropriate level
- Given that the condition has developed over a considerable period of time, the specialist help provided is also likely to take considerable time to work
- Assistance may be given to circumvent the performance problems.

This may be:

i)  on a permanent basis for those who do not wish to remedy the condition;

ii) on a temporary basis to circumvent immediate requirements while the specialist tuition is taking effect. This includes seeking examination concessions where appropriate and necessary for those in this situation and for whom specialist tuition has yet to be fully effective.

On the assumption that possible physical causes are detected and remedied before they can create problems, given the crucial nature of reading and writing for all other intellectual development, great importance should be laid on their development.

The skills and knowledge necessary for their development are well known, as are the ways of helping these develop. It is therefore essential that the development of the ability to read and to convey information in written form is treated as central to intellectual development and forms the core of learning. By this means most problems may be avoided.

However, when problems in these functions do arise, there are two options. If there is insufficient time for appropriate specialist tuition to at least alleviate the problems, then ways may be found to circumvent them—at least until the specialist tuition has taken effect. These circumventions include the use of audio-tape recorders, photocopied notes to overcome difficulties in note-taking, the use of amanuenses in examinations and extra time for examinations.

For adults, there may be good reason for circumventing the problem—at least on a temporary basis and even, in some circumstances, on a permanent one. But especially for children, it is usually judged that, for their future well-being and progress, it is best to develop their fluency in the use of the written language as far as possible and a number of things can help this.

## Implications of the BPsS DECP definition of developmental dyslexia for assessment

It follows from the BPsS DECP definition that the process of deciding whether a person is dyslexic starts with their poor performance in reading and writing. But it can only really be observed over a period of time during which that person exhibits the significant struggle to develop those faculties, despite being provided with adequate opportunity to learn or by an acceptable historical record of that. This requires either great reliance on the recollections of teachers and those affected—not least about whether the latter were committed to learning to read and write! Alternatively, assessment will need to be made over a considerable period of time with careful observation and experiment within appropriate remedial tuition.

In those who have so far failed to develop levels of fluency in reading and writing, both the production of errors and the difficulty in performing the tasks of reading or writing, or both, fluently may be easily observed by using standard performance tests in a diagnostic manner.

In addition, over the period, an apparent difficulty in improving or developing that performance may also be observed. There may also be accompanying emotional or behavioural reaction, although, there may, of course, be other explanations for these.

Establishing the presence of developmental dyslexia in the form of lesser development of brain structure and function might be more problematic in that it might require MRI scanning. Then again, that might be irrelevant in the face of the developmental evidence of Wolpert and of Maguire *et al* (2000).

It might also be unnecessary since 'true dyslexia', as perceived by Snowling, is the one more resistant to remediation and the apparent causes of 'true dyslexia'—in the shape of spoken form deficits and poorer pre-cursor skills and, thus, high risk of later dyslexia—should be evident at the pre-school and Key Stage 1 and so can be relatively easily assessed. The implication is not only that assessment of these should be done at this stage—ages four to six years—but that it should be done **routinely**; and a crucial part of assessment may be of causation.

As for assessment of other conceptions of developmental dyslexia, establishing that an individual has 'Scotopic Sensitivity Syndrome'—or, indeed, any other form of visual difficulty—and minimising it, is likely to remove the reading/spelling problem once they can see what they are looking at. The same is true of all other causes.

For those allegedly suffering 'symptoms' of the 'brain disease' called 'dyslexia', assessment will be of those 'symptoms' using devices such as the Bangor Test to diagnose it. If instead these 'symptoms' are treated as causes and the appropriate remedial action taken, they may find themselves 'cured'.

## Procedures and tests used in assessing reading and spelling

Because the purpose of reading is to acquire information, the fundamental point of assessment is to determine whether you have done so. This normally involves answering questions on what you have read. These answers are often multiple choice, that is, you select what you think is the correct answer from four options. Other tests ask you to supply the answer. Short answers supplied by you need not use the actual words used in the text you read, as long as the meaning is the same. Others again will ask you to do something on the basis of what you have read to see if you understood. Some of these tests will also ask you to read aloud before answering questions.

Other tests of reading are single word recognition tests. These ask you to say what the word is. The mark is given for being able to say the word correctly out loud, even if you don't know what it means. You may know **and recognise** the word and so say it straight away or, if it's less familiar to you, you might be able to work out what it is by guessing on the basis of what it looks like, for example like another word you **do** know or by using phonics to sound it out bit by bit in the hope of recognising the sound of the word which you **do** know.

However, that only works up to a point. For example, you might use this technique to work out the word 'egregious' but have no idea what it means. In that case you may get the mark (depending on the tester) even though you didn't recognise the word in the true sense, and so reading it in the sense of extracting meaning from it is denied you. On the other hand, you may work out the word 'col-o-nel' but have no idea what it means and therefore not know that it's pronounced [kuhnil] in English English and [kurnil] in Scots English. Knowing that would help you to recognise it.

Such tests can therefore be used as word **identification** tests and let the tester know how good you are at working out what words are although you don't get a mark for this. This is important because, in all of these tests, the person who invented the test has chosen a set of words with which he or she is familiar but you might not be. On the other hand, you might know lots of other words of equal difficulty which don't appear in the test. In making the test, the test author will usually pick words with which most people are familiar—usually common and 'concrete' words (describing things)—but to separate out those who know lots of words from those who don't, they use words which are progressively less common and also progressively more abstract (describing feelings or concepts) which fewer and fewer of those taking the test are familiar with.

So the tests might fail to give a good measure of your ability to read—even in the restricted sense of word recognition—on two counts. The set of words chosen by the test author might just not coincide with your personal vocabulary (which just might be better and bigger than the one s/he chose) and it does not account for your ability to work out, at least partly, what the word might be. This latter is a particular issue in dyslexia because the full BPsS definition describes poor performance and a struggle to learn at the single word level, i.e. your recognition vocabulary.

And even if you are not good at working out what words are using the phonics techniques (or even guessing techniques like look and say) (so picking up a few extra marks), this does not mean you are dyslexic in any mysterious sense of that term. It could mean that nobody has taught you those techniques yet, and **that's** why your performance is poor and you're struggling to learn to read. This can be fairly easy checked by having somebody teach you the missing skills and knowledge.

Once you have mastered the basic skills of reading, communicating in the written form of the language and spelling, you will be a competent reader and writer for most everyday purposes. At that point, your reading tactics in particular might change. Because most words are now familiar to you, you will tend not to actually read them but instead look for what are technically called points of critical visual information—the characteristics of a word which identify it as that word and no other—and you will tend to make assumptions about what you are looking at as long as it continues to make sense on the whole.

This is assisted by what is called 'redundancy' in the written text. That means that in most texts you can pick up all of the meaning from reading only about half the words, because you can safely assume that the sentence structure—and so the words you don't read—will be what you might expect from the words you **do** read. You will be able to predict with some accuracy words which you actually didn't read. This can be easily demonstrated from eye movement monitoring when reading and also from 'missing words in a sentence' tests.

There comes a time for all skilled readers when they encounter new, unfamiliar words. This occurs in formal prose such as official letters; for example, from the local council departments, from a solicitor, from the NHS, or from some businesses. It happens to most skilled readers and at that point they resort to the basic 'mechanical' skills they learned at the outset. They may use guessing tactics based on the meaning of the sentence, or they may use phonics—if they know how. As before, if the word is phonically regular, they may be able to pronounce it correctly (but how will they know that?), yet still have no idea of what it means—like 'egregious'—and if it isn't phonically regular, they may have no idea, even, of how to pronounce it (which may not matter until they try to say it to another person who **does** know the word—and then they can look foolish). In either case they may not know what it means or how to pronounce it until somebody else tells them.

Developing reading skills beyond the base level of competence—increasing one's competence in the ranges of register and genre—can be improved immensely by developing one's oral vocabulary and general and specific knowledge, not least by reading widely and discussing what one has read. One's written word 'vocabulary' can also be expanded—for example, to attain the level demanded by one's occupation or higher educational studies—if one possesses the basic skills, including phonics and other tactics, which even skilled readers use to identify unfamiliar words.

## Assessment of adults in reading and spelling

Assessment can be a difficult issue for adults. This is probably because of the negative connotations of the score, and particularly an age score where, as in many tests, these only go up to about fourteen or sixteen years at the most. The reason for this is that there may be an assumption, supported by test norming, that beyond fourteen years people are perfect readers and spellers. This is patently not true. It is more likely that it's much easier to find populations on whom to norm tests in the pre-fourteen school population when whole age groups are available in specific places— schools—as captive audiences.

After this, the populations, even within education, become more diverse (cf. the norms for the Alice Heim series of 'IQ' tests) and after school they become even more so. Because of that increasing diversity, to obtain reasonable adult norms, one would have to sample almost all occupations groups and age *per se* becomes almost irrelevant. This is because, while reading and spelling are developing year on year in school—probably up to the age of fourteen (there are a few exceptions beyond this, such as the old College of Education Entry Test group norms)— thereafter, development of reading and spelling is more likely to be related to the demands of the occupation one finds oneself in. This is similar to development of these skills beyond the mechanical level/expanding one's vocabulary and written communication skills. It may be that for adults, development of literacy beyond the mechanical level is related to the requirements of the occupation to which they gravitate or aspire. It may also be related to the relevant national occupational standards which might in turn be used to derive norms.

It is interesting that the Wide Range of Ability Test (WRAT-3) uses the same relatively short list of words to generate adult norms extending to 77 years of age. It does this by producing a few relatively obscure words (technically low frequency, highly abstract, often phonically irregular words [like egregious, chiaroscuro and synecdoche]) to spread out the respondents at the upper end of the test for all age groups. There is no attempt to correct for educational or occupational advantage.

In assessing reading/spelling difficulties and developmental dyslexia in adults, scores may not matter. The important issue is **how** (and maybe **why**) adults are doing what they are doing and, in particular, the types of mistakes they make. These give clues about whether they are able to use phonics techniques, as well as other techniques, and point to procedures for further investigation of whether they can learn these techniques and so overcome their difficulties. The same clues form the basis of personal learning programmes for those affected.

So, it is possible to use standardised reading and spelling tests successfully with adults—provided these are used diagnostically and ipsatively and all normed or comparative scores are avoided.

# Part 2

# Further reading

## The processes involved in reading

It is easy to forget that there are at least two kinds of reading. The first of these is reading for meaning. This skill extends far beyond reading written or printed words, which are symbolic representations of the sounds of a language. It includes things like reading the signs of oncoming weather, reading the expressions on people's faces, and reading the behaviour of animals— all of which are the acquisition of information or meaning from signs or symbols.

A subset of this kind of reading in the context of verbal— which properly just means 'word' whether spoken or written— language is word recognition, which is a supporting skill for the first kind rather than a separate kind of reading, and the third is word identification, the skill of identifying an unfamiliar word by identifying each of its component parts in turn by the sound each represents, then producing the string or sequence of sounds so identified into a whole which allows recognition of the word-sound so produced. (Note: this does not always work, for example, 'colonel' for a variety of reasons). It may be seen that this is a supporting skill for single word recognition. It should also be noted that the skills and reading behaviours employed in these two types of reading are different. For example, skilled readers do not look at entire words when reading for meaning, but will probably have to do so when attempting to identify an unfamiliar word like 'chiaroscuro'.

Verbal reading for meaning is part of a secondary signalling system (a primary signalling system might be, for example, imitating elephant calls to warn of approaching elephants) which uses **arbitrary** abstract symbols to convey information. These symbols have no intrinsic information value or meaning. They have been evolved over a period of time for use in representing the sounds of the spoken form of the language which was used to convey information long before any form of writing was invented. It is therefore necessary to learn the relationships between symbol and the sounds represented and, ultimately, meaning, in order to become a skilled reader and take part in the transmission of information by this medium.

Because of this, it has to be appreciated that there are **three** major aspects of learning to read. The first of these is 'translating' the symbols on the page back into familiar speech sounds which they were designed to represent—whether or not they make sense at that point (and clearly it would help if they did). This is called 'decoding' by some and is the first stage of a process which should end in word recognition. It may be worth noting that, since if one first learns to produce what one would have otherwise said in the spoken form of the language into a written form which can be transported away from the speaker, and 'listened to' by the intended recipient at a different time and place, it should therefore be easier to learn to read in all senses—'decoding', word identification and comprehension of meaning. To put that another way, if one first learns and understands the point of 'encoding' the spoken form into the written form and how to do it, it may well then be much easier to learn to read in all senses of the word.

The second aspect is recognising familiar words and the third—the real point of reading—is to acquire information and the facility in doing this can be deceptively difficult to measure because English can be as much as 60 per cent redundant. That is, meaning can be conveyed by only 30 per cent of the words in a text.

This is partly because the same idea is elaborated or 're-peated' several times and partly because the text contains operator words (linking or relating words like 'and', 'from', 'the' and 'a', which have little or no meaning by themselves) and lexis words—words which contain meaning. Even among these, there are high information (or unfamiliar) words and low information (familiar) words which are therefore easier to recognise.

Redundancy is, of course, a function of the type of text. So, for example, a novel is about 60 per cent redundant (some current UK tabloid 'newspapers' are probably nearer to 100 per cent!) while scientific or legal text is much less so. **Both types** of the words are necessary for the **accurate** transmission of the information. For an example of the effects, consider Lewis Carroll's *The Jabberwocky* in which nonsense words have been substituted for the **lexis** words, then look at a text from which the **operator** words have been removed. The syntax in the latter will still give some clues to meaning, but much of it is now obscured even if some of it can still be deduced up to a point.

Skilled readers appear to operate a simple process—recognition. However, skilled readers also have recourse to enabling skills for use when things go wrong. The text itself leads the reader to create expectations about what's coming next and redundancy can be a help and a hindrance here. The perceptual processes monitor the succeeding text and the back-up skills are invoked only if the sense or 'story-line' is discontinuous. This is similar to driving up a quiet motorway and suddenly realising that you were 'daydreaming' and have no recollection of the last twenty miles of your journey. The reason is that you were expecting to continue on the motorway for a long while and as long as nothing confounded your expectations (like a sign pointing to someplace which you know is nowhere near your route) then there is nothing to jar the complacency of the monitoring mode of your brain (which may even in the mean time be considering something else.) But sometimes the monitoring isn't skilled enough and so nothing 'jars' and you miss your turning or realise that the car in front is now a bit too close for comfort.

In reading, the skilled reader does not attend to every word and probably would not normally recall a text word for word unless this was also part of the task set. In comprehension tests, the meaning but not the actual wording is usually reported. And when the monitoring of the words is inadequate, misperceptions or miscues occur but it is only when these conflict with the expected meaning that the 'jarring' occurs. These phenomena in reading can be demonstrated by Cloze tests which require the reader to fill in a missing word or phrase from texts.

If the 'jarring' does happen, then the first recourse is usually to whole word identification—and the visual discrimination skills which go with it. Should that fail, then the next recourse is to part-word (morpheme, syllable or letter) which may in turn invoke knowledge of letter/sound relationships (from secondary memory stores) and short-term retention/rehearsal of letter strings (in primary memory) in order to identify the word. Even then it may not be recognised, especially if there is no direct connection from the synthesised word to the known concept (if it **is** known.) This is probably how errors like 'soloyst' occur (perhaps on analogy with 'hoist'?).

And what about the letters 'ui' in the context of different frames, e.g. 'ruin', 'build', 'fruit'? Recognition of these (via stored visual and/or auditory models if present) is a perceptual process. And all depends on the presence of some conceptual structures on which to hang the incoming meaning, otherwise it may be discarded. (Without looking now, can you remember the word at the beginning of this paragraph?)

So, skilled readers take short cuts, **but** they have recourse to a full armoury of skills for use when necessary and there is a fairly large range of skills involved here—all of which have to be mastered on the way to becoming a really skilled reader.

It may be useful at this point to again consider the two aspects of learning to read—and maybe that learning to reading in the sense of 'decoding' the symbols has traditionally been taught the wrong way round; i.e. working from symbol to sound instead of familiar sound expressed as a written symbol. More of that later.

The second aspect of learning to read—in the sense of abstracting information from the test—uses a much greater range of skills and abilities, and it may help to ignore some of the skills developed when learning to 'decode'. What that means is that, unlike in 'decoding', the brain is actively looking for meaning and may be predicting or anticipating yet-to-be-read words in a sentence and so skipping over (i.e. not actually reading) some words and so ignoring decoding—unless of course it ceases to make the sense the reader is being led to expect by the text so far.

In **learning** to read, it is obviously useful to facilitate concept development. (Can it be taught?) The development of spoken forms of storing and communicating these concepts is also very useful, as is the development of whole-word (look and say) **and** part-word identification skills. The skills of visual discrimination are very useful too and usually developed coincidentally in other activities, such as art. The perceptual skills are less often deliberately taught, but it is possible to do so and there are a number of commonly available devices which may be used.

The processes involved in reading

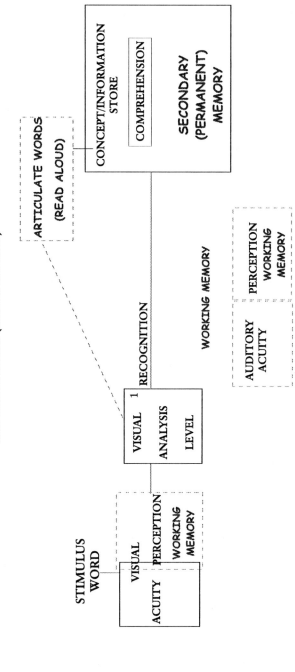

PROCESSES, FUNCTIONS AND SKILLS IN READING
The Direct Route (Skilled Readers)

*The operational pathways are shown by solid lines*

59

and, using the phonics route for identifying unfamiliar words...

## PROCESSES, FUNCTIONS AND SKILLS IN READING

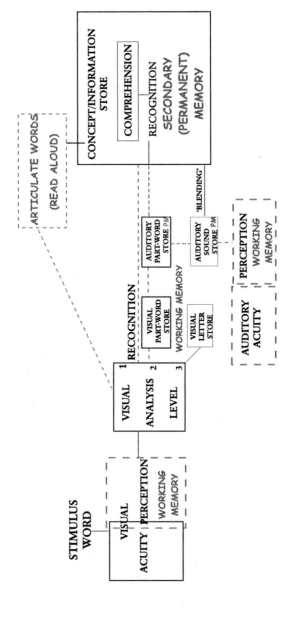

*Similar schematic drawings of operations in spelling are shown in the appropriate section.*

All of these processes are illustrated in the 'model' or 'functional map' of the static processes active in reading and in spelling provided and are shown in such a way that the relationships are evident. This mapping also allows the identification of locations of specific functional deficits or malfunctions so that the effects—and the appropriate remediation—may be easily charted (see pages 59 and 60). This 'model'—which is a relatively simple version, one of many versions of information processing in reading and communicating in writing—shows in simple form the pathways taken by the processing of skilled readers and of less skilled/learner readers.

**Some observations on the processes illustrated in the diagrams on pages 59 and 60**

1. Common forms of temporary, partial deafness, such as 'glue ear' can seriously impair learning to read at the critical stage—as can any uncorrected impaired vision;

2. This scanning is **learned**—probably starting at level 3 on the diagram on page 60 and progressing to level 1 on that diagram. Good readers use level 1 and resort to other levels when necessary. The scanning of unfamiliar words may be unsystematic, cf not-yet-readers and the Pavlidis work;

3. The accurate acquisition (learning) of visual word-forms is critical for spelling (see note 8);

4. Because of the multiplicity of letter/sound, and especially of multiple letter/sounds, a choice has to be made and this may result in the 'blending' of the letters (also a learned skill) into an unrecognised and possibly an unrecognisable 'word';

5. At this point words may be correctly or incorrectly articulated but not comprehended;

6. Concepts are stored and related across many forms—not just verbal;

7. The structures and functions shown in the diagrams in 'black box' form, beloved of cognitive psychologists, may be related directly to the actual structures in the brain;

8.  Production of the visual word form can be on two levels—either direct access to the 'store', or constructed from knowledge of letter/sound relationships. At this lower level the multiplicity of letter/sound relationships again requires choices to be made, resulting in 'phonic' spelling if the **word form** is not known. These are known as 'addressed' spelling and 'assembled' spelling, respectively;

9.  In learning, even if the right word form is taught and practised, it may remain in primary memory and disappear when the exercise finishes—unless it is learned/memorised by either mechanical means, such as making connections with memorable objects, or by mnemonics, or taken into secondary memory by relating it to its meaning (see note 6);

10. The 'rules' for the production of oral forms are not the same as those for producing written forms—so being good at one is not an indicator that one will automatically be good at the other.

Since the ability to use the written form of the language is usually 'mapped on' to pre-existing use of the oral form of the language (which has been, and continues to be, intensively learned and developed by constant use) and depends on there being adequate possession of concepts, ideas or information about things (which form the basis of communication of that information, whether in spoken or written form), these, along with some other things, constitute essential pre-requisites which must be in place before successful 'mapping on' is possible. It is frequently said that the development of these corresponds to stages of maturation—implying physiological maturation.

Apart from the obvious aspects of evolution already discussed, phasing in development is actually more likely to be related to the obvious logical stages. For example, it is obviously the case that the capacity for fine visual discrimination comes before the ability to identify words, although some interaction between the two must continue as the learner learns new words in novel type-faces or forms of print. Since most of the physiological development is in place by the age of nine months, aspects of functional development are unlikely to be determined in a phased fashion controlled by this. They are also unlikely to be related to age—except in a very gross way. The list of pre-requisites includes the following.

*Some of the essential pre-requisites for the successful development of written language handling*

- Adequate neurological structure and function development:
  - Fine visual discrimination and fine auditory discrimination
  - Scanning skills and techniques. Visual analytic skills (using secondary memory 'stores')
  - Blending techniques Visual and aural 'word-form stores'.
- Adequate and controllable motivation and commitment:
  - Attention, habitual arousal state
- Adequate concept formation/intellectual development:
  - cf information obtained from 'intelligence' tests, such as Weschler, BAS and the differences between non-verbal/diagrammatic or 'pure' reasoning and verbal and numerical reasoning—and also the information and vocabulary subtests of WAIS/WISC. Some information obtained by observation of behaviour and discourse
- Adequate oral language handling development:
  - Adequacy of linguistic community/culture (all of which may be restricted:
    - ❖ *Capacity to use and adapt extended forms of spoken language*
  - Sociability/habitual tendency to interact and communicate:
    - ❖ *Adequate vocabulary—'verbally-mediated concept store'*
- Adequate language subskills development:
  - Adequate development of awareness of phonology and skills in phonological analysis and manipulation of pho-

nological entities (letter-sounds, part-word sounds affixes and the like). Awareness of and skilled use of information about the related visual aspects of word-forms.

## Reading difficulties

Many of the points made above are illustrated in the following examples of errors made by poor readers when reading from test passages which require not only accuracy in reading, but also the abstraction of meaning—'comprehension'—from lists of words to be recognised.

### Some typical reading errors

Virtually all of the errors person A made in text reading and single word recognition tasks were misperceptions and frequently mis-articulations, such as 'leads' for 'led', 'appeared' for 'apparently', 'insignificant' for 'insufficient', 'migrate' for 'imitate', 'away' for 'along', 'cologne' for 'colonel' and 'insituation' for 'institution'. He frequently spontaneously corrected several of the words read in error without assistance and when asked to reconsider the remainder, he was able to identify several more.

He also read relatively complex but evidently familiar words, such as 'miscellaneous', 'procrastinate', 'knowledge', 'classification', 'migration', 'originating', 'reappearances' and 'traditional' without hesitation or error, but also showed some tendency to mis-articulate words (such as 'stastistics' for 'statistics') and to add or omit link words, such as 'an' or 'to', apparently at random, when reading from texts.

### A second example of errors produced is:

The errors person B made in the text reading and single word recognition tasks were, for example, 'amusement' for 'amazement', 'place' for 'palace' (both of which were subsequently corrected without assistance), 'bucked' for 'buckled', 'bubbling' for 'bubbles', 'motiousless' for 'motionless', 'smother' for 'shoulder', 'synthetic' for 'systematic', 'sologist' for 'soloist', 'consequence' for 'conscience', 'sensible' for 'susceptible', 'surgical' for 'satirical' and 'biology' for 'biblio- graphy'.

When asked to reconsider words read in error, he was able to identify virtually all of them correctly without assistance. He also read relatively complex but evidently familiar words, such as 'institution', 'classification', 'preliminary', 'prophecy' and 'scintillate' without hesitation or error, but he showed some tendency to add or omit endings such as '-ed', and also link words, such as 'an' or 'to', apparently at random, when reading from texts.

*A third example is as follows:*

Person C reported that when reading text, if the lines were closely spaced, the words appeared to 'jump about'. The errors C made in the text reading and single word recognition tasks were, for example 'expectations' for 'expeditions', 'this will' for 'this is well', 'insignificant' for 'insufficient', 'consistent' for 'conscience', 'sulphurical' for 'sepulchre' and 'homony' for 'homonym'. She also showed some tendency to add or omit word endings and link words, such as 'an' or 'to', apparently at random, when reading from texts.

When asked to reconsider several of the words read in error, and persisting with the accurate identification and subsequent synthesis of constituent sounds of the words, she was able, with some continuing difficulty—generally of mis-articulation followed by an evaporation of confidence, self-consciousness and a resort to inaccurate guessing—to identify some of these correctly, but her use of word identification skills was generally laboured and unskilled.

She also read several relatively complex and evidently familiar words, such as 'systematic', 'classification', 'pneumonia', 'terrestrial', 'preliminary', 'statistics', 'generation', 'rediscovered' and 'ancestors' without hesitation or error.

## The processes involved in communication in writing

The process of communicating in writing starts with the wish to communicate some information and so the concepts are organised, ready for transmission.

In the sound/oral version of verbal communication, the essential base information to be conveyed is produced in the form of 'lexis' or meaningful words selected on the basis of appropriateness for the as accurate as possible conveyance of the 'message'. This might take the initial form of, for example [boy hit man leg]. This basic message is then refined by connecting the lexis words with link or 'operator' words which have little meaning by themselves but, in their proper place, delimit and refine the meaning of the lexis words so that the meaning of the entire message is unmistakable to the receiver. In the preceding example, the message could now be 'The boy hit the man's leg'. It appears that these two stages of the message-creation process are undertaken in sequence by adjacent parts of the language-handling system of the brain.

Further refinement in meaning is achieved by other cues to meaning, such as sound variation (e.g. pitch and tone) and/or accompanying facial expressions and gestures, which can make subtle and not-so-subtle aspects of meaning apparent to the receiver.

It may be helpful to view the production of communication in writing as the 'clothing' of the spoken form in written symbols, with some important exceptions.

In general, the written version of communication follows the same process but, since in written communication the receiver is usually absent, the absence of the opportunity to use these additional spoken or behavioural cues means that the communcator/writer needs to make use of other skills, such as the use of syntax (word order) and conventions of punctuation to achieve the same purpose. Ever more complex concepts can be accurately conveyed by additional use of complex sentence structures, such as embedded clauses.

## The processes involved in spelling

The specific skill of accurate translation of the sound form of words into the correct visual form is at its simplest if the communicator has a good visual word store—perhaps acquired and developed by facility in reading—and a good knowledge of the right visual version to use in particular contexts to convey the desired meaning. It is not long ago since considerable variability in this was acceptable as long as the right meaning was conveyed, but these days, the convention is, in most cases, for only one version to be acceptable.

However, the task is not simply a one-to-one conversion of the sound sequence of a word into its graphic equivalent. The existence of homophones, such as 'bare' and 'bear', only one of which preserves the intended meaning of the entire message, ensures that.

So the speller must **know** the right version to select. That is, the correct visual version of the intended sound and meaning must be available in the communicator's memory for spelling to be other than chance. The value of acquiring the actual visual form of words, as well as the meaning they convey, can now be seen. It is likely that these are acquired after they have been presented a few times in the context of their meaning, which assists their retention. Frequent practice in accurate discrimination of their visual features and pairing with their meaning probably assists their secure storage.

In the absence of such a store of correct visual forms of words whose retrieval may be triggered by the selection of their meaning, spelling becomes a matter of converting the sequence of constituent single letter or letter-group sounds into graphic equivalents. The problem is that there is frequently more than one option and a choice has to be made. The 'rules' of spelling can get one close to the probable right choice, but certainty only comes when one **knows** the right version for the specific circumstances by knowing what the word should look like. That is, the correct version is selected from an adequate visual word store in the memory.

All of these processes are illustrated in the 'model' or 'functional map' of the static processes active in spelling provided, and are shown in such a way that the relationships are evident. This mapping also allows the identification of locations of specific functional deficits or malfunctions so that the effects—and the appropriate remediation—may be easily charted.

This 'model', which is a relatively simple version, one of many versions of information-processing in reading and communicating in writing shows, in simple form, the pathways taken by the processing of skilled readers and of less skilled/learner readers.

## Difficulties in spelling: some typical spelling errors

A's performance resulted in the production of 'Teratore for 'territory', 'apered' for 'appeared', 'explanaytion' for 'explanation', 'Ockashone' for 'occasion', 'neglekted' for 'neglected' and 'genaratone' for 'generation' (but 'particular' and 'regular' were produced correctly, all of which he had read accurately without hesitation in the single word reading test. He also produced 'appresheat' for 'appreciate', 'eckwiley' for 'equally', 'indeviduel' for 'individual', 'enfuseastik' for 'enthusiastic' and 'sethisient' for 'sufficient'.

*A second example of spelling is:*

B's attempts at spelling produced 'sucer' for 'saucer', 'ANgle' for 'angel', 'upeared' for 'appeared', 'cannier' for 'canary', 'atraca...' for 'attractive' and 'inmargin' for 'imagine', all of which he had read without hesitation in the single word reading test. He also produced 'scite' for 'sight', 'brout' for 'brought' and 'mined' for 'mind', and observed that he knew these were incorrect but could not identify the actual errors, but also produced 'large', 'mouth', 'dream', 'year' and 'sooner' correctly, without hesitation.

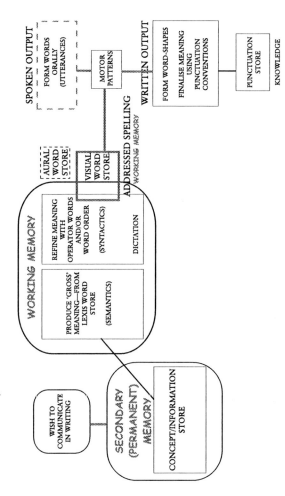

## PROCESSES, FUNCTIONS & SKILLS IN COMMUNICATING IN WRITING

WISH TO COMMUNICATE IN WRITING

**SECONDARY (PERMANENT) MEMORY**

CONCEPT/INFORMATION STORE

**WORKING MEMORY**

PRODUCE 'GROSS' MEANING—FROM LEXIS WORD STORE (SEMANTICS)

REFINE MEANING WITH OPERATOR WORDS AND/OR WORD ORDER (SYNTACTICS)

DICTATION

AURAL WORD STORE

VISUAL WORD STORE

ADDRESSED SPELLING WORKING MEMORY

**SPOKEN OUTPUT**

FORM WORDS ORALLY (UTTERANCES)

MOTOR PATTERNS

**WRITTEN OUTPUT**

FORM WORD-SHAPES

FINALISE MEANING USING PUNCTUATION CONVENTIONS

PUNCTUATION STORE

KNOWLEDGE

The diagram above shows—from left to right along the solid lines—the main processes in addressed spelling. That on overleaf shows the main processes in assembled spelling—using 'phonics' phonological analysis of the sound model.

Dyslexia is not a brain disease

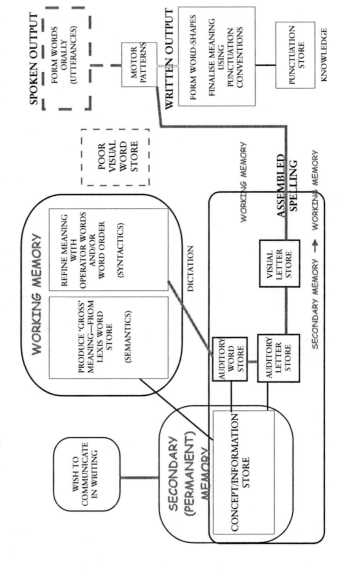

PROCESSES, FUNCTIONS & SKILLS IN COMMUNICATING IN WRITING

70

*A third example of this is:*

C's productions in the test of spelling were, for example, 'InSTartution' for 'institution', 'genuwin for 'genuine', 'SiStamatic' for 'systematic', 'Tartory' for 'territory' and 'Ecencheal' for 'essential', all of which she had read without hesitation in the single word reading test. She also produced 'Silppare' for 'slippery', 'sumalur' for 'similar', 'pernament' for 'permanent', 'safishant' for 'sufficient', 'infuseastic' for 'enthusiastic' (both evidently as she pronounced them), 'espeshley' for 'especially' and 'missalaneous' for 'miscellaneous' in a formal single word spelling test.

When asked to try the techniques of repeating the words aloud while converting their constituent sounds into letter-form, it was evident that C had considerable difficulty in producing accurate articulation of the words concerned. Her mis-articulations were apparently related to those produced during her attempts to identify unfamiliar words by accurate analysis and subsequent 'blending' of their constituent parts when reading.

## Spelling problems: some solutions

Spelling is the production or 'clothing' of words in the spoken form of a language into a written or printed form of symbols (letters) which represent them and therefore allows the message produced by the speaker to be transported to a recipient in another time or place.

Reading is the act of then 'decoding' these symbols to gain access to the message. The processes and skills of reading are therefore determined by the process of 'encoding' or spelling. Spelling is not a generative process. It is one of remembering precisely the way in which any specific word was 'clothed' in letters—and this may have changed over time. There are therefore no rules of spelling, but there are aids to remembering how a word is constructed and this is helped by there being some consistency—and also some conventions—which have brought many originally differently constructed words together in a similar way. The conventions are those of the writing (spelling) process and, while in any language there are many consistencies in the way in which specific speech sounds are 'encoded into written or printed form, in the English language in particular—because of the plethora of words from other languages which have been incorporated for historical reasons—an often large range of ways in which individual speech sounds can be produced in written form has developed.

Successful performance in spelling is often restricted to words which are evidently very familiar—that is, for which the visual image was available for recall. The process by which spelling is performed in this way is by the direct route from memory store of the visual image of the word being spelled, via the motor plans for appropriate movement of the hand in drawing the letters or words. It is known as 'addressed' spelling where direct use of the visual image is made.

Skilled spellers therefore most probably use visual images of words stored in their memory when spelling words and this avoids all of the problems, such as the mismatch of the look and the sound of words, inherent in various ways in the English language.

If these visual images are not available or not very clear in the memory, it becomes necessary to resort to other techniques—most often that known as 'phonological' or phonic spelling (that is, a direct transcription of the constituent sounds of the word into the letters commonly used to represent these sounds), but sometimes the techniques and the information they use become mixed up during use with even more unfortunate results.

Examples of these might be similar to those recently produced by one young person who used: 'brot' for 'brought', 'polisea' for 'policy', 'siht' for 'sight' (yet 'might' correctly spelled), 'libary' for 'library', 'logh' (the spurious 'h' added as an afterthought) for 'lodge' and 'deirect' for 'direct', all of which are phonically accurate.

However, attempts to attribute causation to such productions are confounded because the same person can produce words of equal complexity which are evidently very familiar, such as 'final' and 'circus' correctly but in the latter case after spontaneous correction from 'curcus'.

The form of errors like these suggests that they were produced on the basis of uncertainty of visual forms and, oddly enough, that can actually be caused or made worse by inadequate reading behaviours, such as poor use of word identification techniques of analysis and synthesis (which is best for a number of reasons if it includes simultaneous enunciation of the analysed 'bits' while synthesising these aloud into the recognisable word sound). That forces the speller to be over-reliant on sound 'models', which is often made worse by interference in the 'pure' process by an erratic awareness and use of at least part of the correct visual forms, or assumption of these by analogy with other known similar-looking or sounding words. This is known as 'assembled' spelling, which produces 'phonic' spelling and up to about 100 years ago was acceptable in polite society but is not now. It also has its problems.

Spelling, using the technique of conversion of sounds to words, sound by sound, depends firstly on the accuracy of the sound model and is, thereafter, a probabalistic process, since, in the English language, there are frequently several options for production of sounds in letter form. The ultimate decision about correctness requires resort to a mental store of visual forms of words which are largely acquired in the process of reading and in practising spelling. Unskilled readers are likely to be denied adequate development of this store of information.

The process can also be 'assisted'—and also made worse— by use of 'spelling rules'. These 'rules' can provide guidance on how a word should look, but they are often actually rules about how the word changes its **sound** and, worse, they are not consistent, i.e. they do not always apply. There are many 'exceptions' and the reasons are not usually logical. Because of that, spelling by this method is not only probababalistic but also conditional and inconsistently so—which does not help anyone and confuses those sharp enough to look for consistencies and logic. For example, it is often said that a 'vowel' coming after a double consonant is short, but if the preceding consonant is single, the vowel is long—as, for example in 'rudder' and 'ruder'.

The first problem is that the learner speller has to learn new terminology (like 'consonant') and the second is that the statement is only partly accurate. The reality is that the 'u' in 'ruder' is 'held' (the sound is made for a longer period of time) longer but *it is also a different sound*! The vowel sound in 'rudder' is [uh] while in 'ruder' it is [oo]. It isn't just 'held' for longer.

The point of that information is that if one is spelling these words primarily by listening to the string or series of sounds which make up a word and writing them down one by one, to form the word (phonetic spelling), the actual 'rule' is that where the same letter ('u') is used, if it makes the sound [oo], the consonant following it will be a single one whereas if it makes the sound [uh], two consonants of the same kind will follow it.

So, knowing the 'rules' for spelling can be beneficial but cannot be the complete answer—and may lead to confusion if not known perfectly.

**Some suggestions for spelling development**

Successful addressed spelling requires a memory storage of the accurate, complete visual image of words. This is acquired both by using the analytic techniques of identification of unknown words and by practising this technique on known words.

The 'synthesis' or saying aloud of the string of bit-words into the whole word-sound not only aids the potential recognition of the word-sound as a known word, it is also in a way 'spelling'. Therefore practising spelling by breaking the word-sound into a string of sounds—preferably to the accompaniment of a 'beat' for each syllable—is also a powerful aid to spelling because it, too, helps the memorability of the string of sounds and its retention in working memory.

Practising spelling in this way is a good way to learn to be a good speller—up to a point. The other requirement is to recall just how the sounds **in this word** are represented by letters or lettergroups. That comes from careful analysis of the visual and sound parts of the word together when reading, or exercising the skills of word identification. Frequent practice in the identification of unfamiliar words, as well as exploration of the constituent visual and aural parts of known, complex words—using the subskills of visual and phonological analysis and subsequent re-synthesis of words suggested—for the development of reading skills should also assist in consistent and accurate acquisition of the visual forms of these words for retrieval for use in spelling. The information obtained in this way should be used in intensive practice of the production of the correct versions of words about whose spelling the learner is uncertain until this becomes automatic.

There are a number of computer programs which can be used to explore the ways in which words can be segmented into syllables, part-words or even individual letters in the manner suggested. Some of these will allow the words to be broken up into whatever suits the learner, and this is important because whatever the learner is comfortable with is the way they will best remember the bits which constitute the word. Other programs will not allow this but may nevertheless assist in the process of visual and aural analysis and so assist in the memorability of the bits produced.

As with most things in life, practice makes perfect, so once the constituent underpinning skills have been mastered, the accurate production of the actual forms of the words, using a combination of rehearsal of the accurate sound version of a word together with accurate recall of its visual form, developed from the exercises suggested, should be practised intensively and progress checked frequently but sympathetically, with constructive evaluation and assistance provided for the achievement of improvement in performance.

### Spelling—writing as you speak, maybe?

> *'Aoccdrnig to rscheearch at Cmabrigde Uinervtisy, it deosn't mttaer inwaht oredr the ltteers in a word are, the only iprmoetnt thing is tahtthe frist an lsat ltteer be at the rghit pclae. The rset can be a total mses and you can still raed it wouthit porbelm. This is bcuseae the human mind deos not raed ervey lteter by istlef, but the wrd as a wlohe.'*

This passage was distributed in an email to his colleagues by an 'expert' in adult literacy who really ought to know better than suggest, as he did, that the conclusion of the research—cited in the passage above—was wrong (in case you really can't read it, it says that research at Cambridge has shown that readers look at only the beginnings and ends of words so the letter order between these can be jumbled and it makes no difference to their ability to read).

I don't know this research but from other research I do know of, I think it's probably true—of **skilled** readers! However, it's not so far removed from the onset and rime aspect of phonics that some learner readers use/are taught (maybe). The research may actually have import for the way learner readers are taught (although I think not, unless it's to draw attention to the onset and rime tactic) or the implications for learning to spell via being 'caught' from the act of reading and that reminded me of the old chestnut, 'is spelling caught or taught?' (a false distinction, by the way).

That led me to thinking about learning to spell and the issue of whether spelling is a matter of writing down what you would otherwise have said and, if not, what more is there to it? Writing what you would otherwise have said will produce 'phonic' or 'phonetic' spelling—some of which will be 'errors'. That's because English is not phonetic.

So what else do you need to know or be able to do to produce 'correct' spelling? 'Correct' spelling is a social phenomenon. To be acceptable (and to avoid being thought to be 'thick'), it is necessary to produce 'correct' spelling—spelling which conforms to the currently ordained orthography (I say 'current' because it wasn't always like that). Somebody somewhere in a position of appropriate 'authority', for whatever reason, decided that only one version of a written form of a word is acceptable in polite society. Andy Ellis, in his book *Reading, Writing and Dyslexia*, gives examples of well-meaning lexicographers actually (wrongly) changing the spelling of words so that they conform to the spelling of other, totally unrelated words. Noah Webster did the same—and maybe even Sam Johnson too—when compiling their dictionaries.

Putting the rights and wrongs of that aside for the moment, how can you ensure that your spelling is 'correct'? Clearly, writing down the sounds of what you would say is insufficient. That's because in English, particularly, there are very often options for expressing sounds in letter form. So that leaves you with options—just like spellcheckers do!

Maybe you could teach the optional ways of expressing the sounds of the spoken language and the probabilities of the appearance of each in specific words. There are several teaching programmes on the market which do exactly that. You will find a short list in Martyn Long's paper and also her own version in Diane McGuinness's book and related work on spelling.

In that context, there may be merit in considering at length why reading is normally taught before writing and spelling. After all, logic might suggest that, since most of us normally develop some fluency in the spoken language pre-school, the next step would be to learn how this is converted into the written form. Doing that makes the reasons why we are doing it—to 'speak' to somebody in another time or place—clear, and almost automatically shows the learner how and why to read.

That's one possibility—just like the 'phonics' technique is only one tactic for reading at the level of word identification. The essence of spelling in a conglomerate language like English is that to do it 'correctly', you **must** know what the word looks like. There is no way round it, which means that, in spelling, you must be able to retrieve the visual/written form of the word from long-term memory. This, of course, assumes that they are in there—and stored in such a way as to be readily retrievable when required. If not, you have to resort to other tactics—like converting the sounds of words you can 'hear' in your head into letters which clearly **do** represent those sounds—i.e. 'phonic spelling'.

That brings into question issues of how the accurate visual forms of words are acquired/learned, how they are stored and how they are made accessible when required—all of which are interlinked but are big issues in their own right in the realms of memory studies. For example, spelling 'rules' are not really rules at all, because the process is not generative. They are instead ways of facilitating memory; specifically, aids to retrieving the actual visual form (if stored)—i.e. what it actually looks like, in spite of what it sounds like—of the word to be spelled. And so we get back to reading solely by looking at the beginning and end of words.

How do we acquire the visual form of words, if not taught to write down our spoken communication before being taught how to read—and/or before learning the options and probabilities for writing spoken word sounds in letter form? Can it be incidental to reading? Given that reading is primarily for the purpose of acquiring meaning and that skilled readers therefore do not attend to every detail of the words they are reading, and that learner readers use a number of other techniques—including guessing from context or accompanying pictures and not actually reading some words at all—what opportunity is there for them to acquire and store the complete and accurate visual form of words?

If they don't, how **do** they acquire the visual form? One common way is by rote learning of lists of unrelated words to be produced later in response to 'dictation' of these in a spelling test for marks out of ten. This is known to be inefficient—not least because the storage is out of context of the meaning of the word (meaningfulness is by far the most powerful facilitator of storage in long-term memory). It's also the case that once used, such rote learning tends to be discarded from long-term memory precisely because it's no longer of any practical value—it has no real meaning or further value for the individual once they have taken the test.

So, how can we improve spelling? Is it a matter of using the principles outlined above and all the tactics too? To begin to answer that we need to consider the processes involved in spelling—cognition, information-processing in the proscribed forms and concepts of cognitive psychology and memory function.

## Exploring further the concept of developmental dyslexia: What do you mean 'Developmental'?

Because there are several interpretations of the term 'developmental' in this context, it may be worth exploring just what it means here. 'Acquired' as in acquired dyslexia is self-evident. 'Developmental' in this context is a bit more open to interpretation because it can have several meanings—just to add to the confusion. Cause and effect in acquired dyslexia are obvious. There is damage to the relevant areas of the brain and the resultant impairment of language use are characteristic of the locus of damage (examples of these are found on pages 80 and 81).

Nobody asks, 'is this dyslexia?' The dysfunction of the formerly normally functioning lexical/language-handling system is obvious from the errors made. This dyslexia is usually the least of the patient's worries—at first anyway—and damage resulting only in dyslexia is very rare indeed. Developmental dyslexia is different.

'Developmental' can be active or passive. It can mean the 'natural'/incidental evolution of the relevant brain structure and function or it can mean the deliberate, intentional development, as in the course of teaching. It can apply to structural development, which is affected by experience and use (see Maguire *et al*, 2000; Wolpert, 1991). It can mean function development generally—also evolved by experience and use, or development of the language handling systems (developed by experience and use, not least by socio-cultural factors), especially for the precursor skills, knowledge and motivation

Using the written language is not a naturally occurring phenomenon. It is a learned facility. If nothing were done to learn it, it would not appear and would make little difference to the individual's fundamental ability to make his/her way in the world other than in the increasingly information-based society in which we now live. It is therefore not developmental in the same way as, for instance, vision or walking upright are developmental. It is developed, that is, it can be taught, learned and deliberately improved and fine tuned by formal or informal, intentional or incidental tuition and/or learning.

## Acquired Dyslexia: Examples of error types

Wernicke's area is the area of the left hemisphere temporal lobe of the brain. This area is thought to be the main 'marshalling' area for lexical words— those words which carry meaning.

Damage to this area produces loss of meaningful content words in utterances in the spoken form and sentences in the written form, for example:

**Wernicke's area damage – spoken output**

'before I was the one here, I was over in the other one. My sister had the department in the other one.'

**Patient describing where he lived before his accident**

'the telephone man in the process of describing the existence and spectatorship of .... in the West Country. The tunnership were ... the for utteridge of the er .... vessel. It really is what's in it's front tyre.'

**patient describing a drawing of a telegram boy standing by a grass verge, holding his bicycle the front wheel of which is lying on the ground.**

**Wernicke's area damage – reading**

Table read as **Chair**

Small read as **Little**

Antique read as **Vase**

Canary read as **Parrot**

Gnome read as **Pixie**

Note that the reader appears to recognise the meaning but access to the actual word is apparently denied.

## Acquired Dyslexia: Examples of error types (contd)

### Broca's area damage – spoken output

Broca's area is an area to the front of the left hemisphere temporal lobe of the brain. This area is thought to be the main area for the adding lexical words – those words which carry little or no meaning by themselves but further delineate or 'disambiguate' the meaning of the lexical content to make complete utterances or sentences.

Damage to this area produces 'telegrammatic' speech or writing in which the basic content is present but the fine nuance is lost. for example:

'Go....New York'

Patient describing journey from his home to the hospital in New York where he now is.

1. 'Girl is...flower...the woman!
2. 'The teacher is...the girl...giving it...teacher'
3. 'The girl is...flower...teachers'

three different patients describing a picture of a little girl giving flowers to her teacher

### Broca's area damage – reading

Put five shillings on a good horse

read as

Five bob...best horse

Patient reading a text. Note the retention of basic meaning but loss of accurate meaning.

### Is this where the notion of dyslexia as a brain disease comes from?

Developmental dyslexia was first postulated because there was no damage and no obvious cause, giving rise to speculation of 'minimal brain damage' (MBD). Later, this was extended to cases where individuals had developed other intellectual abilities to a high level so the cause must be specific learning difficulty. The possible reasons for failure to develop the complex skills and knowledge required in learning to read and write were—and continue to be—largely ignored. All that can be seen is the poor performance and, upon good investigation, the struggle to improve.

Especially in the context of other intellectual/academic ability the 'most important' question is, 'Is this dyslexia?' This is a loaded question. It implies both 'is dyslexia **causing** this?' and that it can't possibly be due to normal causes.

## The possibility of biological development failure in structure and/or function

### The interactions in reading ability between demand, use, subserving brain structure and function: leading to fallacies of causation

It is well known and documented in neuropsychology that the neural pathways, from birth, evolve, expand and even in some situations, atrophy, in response to the use, or lack of it, which is made of them. Some such brain systems will, under normal conditions, inevitably develop fully to undertake the basic needs of the organism. Others, which subserve certain activities that require to be learned and may or may not be, i.e. the use of language, and which may or may not evolve partially or fully if use—especially extended use made by, for example, higher academic learning or occupation—is not made of them. This may in turn depend on the demands made of the situations, such as that of advancement in occupation, in which they exist.

There has, however, been a tradition in the study of developmental dyslexia of accepting evidence—initially from post-mortem studies and latterly from brain scans—that some related structure or function is not fully developed and that this, therefore, is the root cause of the poor reading* problems/developmental dyslexia. This may be especially true when the under-developed or 'unusual' structure or function is located in, and specific to, the language-handling neural pathway systems of the brain. In this case it is said to be evident that the problem is a **developmental** one and, moreover, a **biological** developmental anomaly. Some even claim that dyslexia is the **cause** of this biological underdevelopment.

There have been many instances of this. Geschwind and others in 1972 postulated that, in dyslexics (for whom the evidence of dyslexia as distinct from 'ordinary poor readers' is very debatable), the problem was an underdeveloped left temporal planum. In 1981, Pavlidis postulated that developmental dyslexia, defined in accordance with a 'wastebasket' paradigm (it's

---

\*    Here used to mean all aspects of the use of the written form of the language

83

not this, nor this, so it must be whatever is left), was caused by erratic, unsystematic eye movements when scanning text—an underdevelopment of function. There have been, and still are, others seen on fMRI scans of the relevant areas of the brain during experiments which require the subject to read or write while being scanned.

In such cases, the evidence is gathered either at the time when the sufferer is dead, or still in the throes of exhibiting poor skills development and before any attempt has been made to improve their learning. And that's the key. No account is taken of the fact that these are learned abilities and that structure and function are known to develop in accordance with learning and use and so would be developed as a result of that learning. Apart from Pavlidis's apparent overlooking of the nature of looking behaviour in this context—known to optometry but not always taken into account in the psychology of reading—it can be shown that the reason for the inadequate saccadic movements of these 'dyslexics' is **because they haven't yet learned how to read.** The same is likely to be true of other claimed biological structural and/or functional failures, because they measure these only at the time when the sufferer is exhibiting problems and apparently not again after the individual concerned has been successfully taught to read.

The work of Vellutino, cited by Snowling, led her to suggest that 'true dyslexics' are only those relatively few who are resistant to remedial tuition; there is some evidence to suggest that the reason for that might well be that they have come to the learning situation poorly equipped for such learning, i.e. lacking the precursor skills, knowledge and perhaps motivation, often because of a socio-cultural background which does not value such development and therefore takes no steps to foster it.

The work of Maguire et al (2000), on the relevant brain structure and function evolution of taxi drivers in right hemisphere spatial orientation activities, underlines the basic proposition, of which basic psychology is replete with evidence, that neural pathways evolve in response to use—some of which is in response to the demands of life in all its ramifications. Surely learning how to use the written form of the language can't be different. Surely the relevant structures and functions will be seen in subsequent fMRI scans to have evolved after successful remedial tuition. That's a testable hypothesis...

## Isolating the developmental dyslexic from other poor readers: the research evidence

The factor used to distinguish generally backward readers (GRR) from specific reading retardation (SRR) is IQ. They are otherwise undistinguishable unless one takes those in Vellutino's (1996) study VLG group (those with the least good response to intervention) as the defining characteristic. If so, **this** is the defining characteristic—poor development of precursor skills and knowledge—and there can be 'normal' reasons for it. Snowling suggests that these might be the 'true dyslexics'—those particularly resistant to improvement given remedial tuition.

However, Snowling (2000) also cites research which indicates that 'true dyslexics' differ on 'cognitive profile'. In practice, the dimensions of this cited—poor phonological awareness and related phonological skills, verbal short-term memory, and slowness in rapid naming—are all what Goswami calls precursor skills. These are the abilities which children bring to school with them on first entry and the variability across individuals is enormous. They are also abilities that can be developed in pre-school years, influenced by their 'environment' which includes social, cultural and other aspects as well as the physical environment.

In addition, Share et al (1987) and Shaywitz et al (1992) did not find that discrepancy-defined 'dyslexics' had an especially poor prognosis. Instead, there was some evidence that SRR did better than GRR. The differences in progress made by these groups not only varied over time but sometimes one and sometimes the other made better progress. Ultimately the only consistent difference between the two groups was the difference in 'IQ'. This contradicts any suggestion that 'dyslexics' somehow have different brain arrangements or functioning, or think differently from the rest of us—or indeed are the only group suffering from dyslexia.

Moreover, Stanovitch et al have shown that the correlation between IQ and reading is—for what it's worth—at best only

0.3. That is, only about 9 per cent of the variance is shared, which does not imply causation. Snowling interprets this as the final, conclusive evidence that there is no validity in the 'discrepancy' model for identifying or diagnosing dyslexia. In other words, as research by the BPsS DECP has also concluded, IQ has little or nothing to do with dyslexia. In addition, also contrary to popular mythology—based on the usual list of 'symptoms' or 'indicators' of dyslexia—Rutter and Yule (1975), and others, showed a different picture.

Specifically, generally poor readers (the GRR group) show more neurological 'soft' signs, such as movement disorders and clumsiness, as well as more neurological impairments, such as epilepsy, than the specific reading retarded (SRR) group. In addition, the SRR group were better at the 'finger agnosia' test, (a test often used as a sign or symptom of dyslexia), at sentence memory and at object naming. Both groups show raised incidence of indicators of onset of speech, of speech and language problems and of incidence of this in the family. The groups did, however, differ in respect of SRR having more complex language use, which is consistent with their higher IQ.

## Distinguishing the dyslexic from other poor readers: further exploration of the distinguishing characteristics of developmental dyslexia

Essentially, the BPsS DECP definition of developmental dyslexia is a descriptive term for extraordinary difficulty in developing appropriate levels of fluency in the skills of reading and writing and/or an incomplete development of these. It is a description of the observed situation—the production of errors and extraordinary difficulty in improving performance. The essential difference between dyslexics and other poor readers is that, for the latter, the development of the faculties of reading and communicating in the written form of the language is, or should be, relatively easily overcome. According to recent research, the distinguishing characteristic of developmental dyslexia might be its resistance to intervention with remedial tuition—and this, in turn, may be because of poor development of precursor skills and knowledge prior to starting to learn to read. There are many possible reasons for that.

Some, however, assert that there are other differences. Those who conceive dyslexia as a 'different way of thinking' caused by 'developmental miswiring of the brain', also assert that dyslexics are **unable** to perform many of the constituent tasks of reading, writing and spelling, as well as several other unrelated behaviours **because** they think or 'process information' differently from the rest of us. This assertion can be tested relatively easily—and in the course of this, it is as well to remember that there is a big difference between 'can't', 'don't' and even, for some, 'won't'. Some may choose not to try to overcome the problem, sometimes in the belief that it can't be overcome.

Most learner readers, including dyslexics, 'don't' precisely because they haven't yet learned to, but evidence on the effects of intervention (e.g. Vellutino, 1996) show that they can and do improve. The Dyslexia Institute has similar evidence derived from investigation of the effects of tuition. Dyslexics **can** read, write and spell to a fair extent. The extent to which they can do this will vary in accordance with a fair number of factors. These are listed on page 63. They **may** make more errors more frequently than some other groups of learners. However, unlike in acquired dyslexia, the errors made by developmental dyslexics are no different from those made by anyone else—especially those made by other poor readers—and all might be attributable to normal causes.

So, if dyslexics are no different from other poor readers in respect of the errors they make or the difficulties they have, in what way **are** they different? The term 'dyslexia' is said by some to be applicable only when the struggle to develop appropriate levels of fluency is seen in those who have developed their other intellectual abilities 'normally'. In such cases, the problem is also called specific learning difficulty. That's because inadequate development of appropriate levels of fluency in the use of the written language may be the **only** difficulty they have. This is an interesting issue since, given that reading and writing are a means of conveying information, this specificity implies that other intellectual development, i.e. in academic subjects, is unaffected. This is probably because the information required for such development is acquired and transmitted in ways other than those of the written language. However, it is likely that this 'blocked channel' of information conveyance is nonetheless a restricting factor on such development. Nevertheless, because of this, the poor performances in reading and writing are said to be *unexpected* and this is enough for some to say that **this unexpectedness** is the distinguishing characteristic of developmental dyslexia.

However, limiting the label of dyslexic to this group may be quite wrong. This is because, as recent research shows, the nature of their difficulties in reading, writing and spelling, and the things which cause them, are no different from the same difficulties experienced by those whose other intellectual development so far is also restricted. Unfortunately, this group is usually but wrongly perceived to be intellectually unable to do any better than they do. It can be argued instead that, given access to information in the written form, intellectual development would follow. The restricted general intellectual development of this group may therefore be a consequence of their restricted fluency in the use of the written language. In other words, the difference between them and those whose restriction is only in use of the written language is that the latter have found ways of circumventing the problem and acquiring information by other means and the others haven't yet been helped to do that. This is relatively easy to demonstrate.

It is also said by some to be necessary to reject poor readers who have a history of absence from school or are judged to lack the intellectual ability to learn to read or to go beyond the modest level they have attained so far. In such cases, they say, the poor reading is only to be expected. Others go even further. The term 'dyslexia' is said by them not to be applicable when the cause of the problems is, for example, inadequate IQ or inadequate schooling—as implied in the extended definition above—and obvious visual or hearing difficulties should also be excluded. So that, too, is only to be expected. But is it?

It may be quite wrong to deny that those for whom these things are the cause are also dyslexic as defined above. It may be wrong because these situations can produce exactly the same

effect or condition described by the BPsS DECP c
These criteria for rejection have formed the basis of s(
definitions of developmental dyslexia—essentially 'wa
definitions—in which, after rejection of the obvious causes, one
is left with the answer. For some, this 'answer' has been the sup-
position of some mysterious 'neural' cause and probably also led
to the specific learning difficulty proposition as the exclusive
definition of developmental dyslexia. So, can these causes be
legitimately excluded?

The suggestion that inadequate IQ is a basis for excluding
poor readers from being dyslexic—a variant of the specific
learning difficulty argument—is debatable. How much IQ is
necessary to be able to learn to read at the 'mechanical' level of
word identification? What constitutes 'intelligence' and what
constitutes 'adequate' in this context are seldom addressed but
really need to be if we are to safely discount this as the cause. At
the level of single word recognition or identification—or 'decoding'—it is likely to be minimal and specific.

Current research shows that learning to read requires specific knowledge and skills, collectively known as precursor skills.
In recent years, most research has acknowledged phonological
awareness and the application of related skills—and perhaps of a
similar kind—as the 'intelligence' needed. So the sort of ability
assessed by IQ tests is probably minimal, and related to specific
things, such as vocabulary and general knowledge. The ability to
read and write beyond the 'mechanical' coding/decoding level is
dependent on the 'higher IQ' of appropriate levels of relevant
knowledge of the subject matter of the communication (and that
applies to you right now in reading this). If there is little or nothing to convey, the system for conveying it will be appropriately
undeveloped, but that is well beyond the scope of the BPsS
DECP and most other definitions.

It is therefore unsafe to exclude poor readers from being
dyslexic on the basis of inadequate IQ before we have clearly
identified what this is and how much is necessary. Poor reading
performance together with extraordinary struggle to improve,
which is the apparent result of prolonged absence from school,
is also excluded from being labelled dyslexia. The implication is
that these poor performances, too, are only to be expected,

unlike those for whom there is no evidence of difficulty in developing appropriate levels of performance in other intellectual functions. However, that, too, might be debatable—not least because of the possible reasons for absence. These include illness and the social and emotional reactions to failing at school which can themselves obstruct learning. Those things which cause absence from school, as well as the absence itself, may be the cause of other things, such as poor development of subskills, for example phonological skills or memory operations. But presence in school does not guarantee the acquisition of those.

The provision of teaching or opportunity to learn or even being taught is not the same as learning. Most of us know from experience in one or both directions that it is possible to be there when teaching is taking place, yet learning is not. There are many reasons for this, not least the motivation to learn—possibly the most crucial factor of all—which varies according to the interest we have in learning whatever it is that we have the opportunity to learn. Then there are all the other factors involved in learning, any of which can seriously obstruct it. Not least of these is that, for five year olds, it is usually somebody else's idea to learn to read and not necessary for practical purposes at that point. The necessary motivation, therefore, may well be lacking. So might pre-school development of precursor skills, perhaps because of socio-cultural factors.

It may be, for example that the observed extraordinary difficulty in developing the precursor awareness of phonology of the spoken language and application of related skills could be the result of difficulty in comprehending what is required and that, in turn, could be the consequence of a failure to present learners with the information they need in a way which is comprehendable—either generally or to them personally—since learning and memory are idiosyncratic. Performance is largely determined by the way what is to be learned is presented for learning, thus enabling acquisition and retention of information and, consequently, when required, retrieval and output. It is unlikely that those affected do not have the mental ability to understand.

It may be that a learner's learning style or mind-set makes it difficult for them to take in what they are being presented with because it is not within their current experience or not presented in a way that makes sense to them; this could depend on what they already know or don't know. Some may be attempting to force a logic which doesn't exist on spelling. Even assuming the factors essential for learning are all in place and positive, development of the skills of reading and communicating in the written form of the language requires stepwise or stage-related development of the subskills, i.e. particular aspects of memory or those of analysis of the phonology of the language, which enable the development of these high-level abilities. Evidence of the opportunity to learn these and, more importantly, of the learner's positive engagement, is hard to find when, typically, assessment for dyslexia is made several years later. Absence from school is therefore not so easily dismissed as a possible explanation either.

In addition, one might also argue that the other causes—visual, hearing and memory problems and other factors—are also only to be expected in the same way as school absence and inadequate intelligence, once we know that they are present. A real problem here is that these physical function problems are not easily, and therefore not usually, detected, although this can be because we don't bother screening for them. However, one **can** observe potential **causes** of dyslexia (see the list on pages 41/42, although their presence alone shouldn't be construed as proof of dyslexia). If these other features are present, they are difficulties in their own right, not manifestations of a developmental failure called dyslexia.

**What is not dyslexia?**

Some people assert instead that dyslexia is a mysterious ailment, supposed by proponents of this conception to be at the neural level, a 'miswiring of the brain' or abnormal—but not necessarily less able—way of thinking about things, which is the cause of the struggle to learn to read and write and a few other things besides. This supposed abnormal way of thinking is sometimes referred to by its proponents as information-processing, but is very different from the scientific use of that term by cognitive psychologists, and the entire set of assertions is a radically different conception from that defined by the BPsS DECP.

Proponents further assert that this ailment can manifest itself as disorganised thinking and behaviour, particular kinds of memory dysfunction and/or visual or hearing difficulties, such as apparently seeing things back to front or being unable to differentiate left from right. In practice, most of these 'symptoms' are actually potential causes of dyslexia as defined by the BPsS DECP. Rigorous investigation can normally separate real cause from actual effect. This is critical for the effectiveness of tuition.

## The effects of being dyslexic

Developmental dyslexia does **not** prevent learning, but the things which cause dyslexia **do** obstruct learning to read and write. That, in turn, may obstruct learning. Especially in the context of academic development, where most of the information provided for learning—and sought as proof of learning, in the form of examinations and tests—is in the written form of the language, possession of appropriate levels of fluency in reading and writing, and in working with numbers are crucial. Reading, writing and working with numbers at an appropriate level of fluency, that is, such that they do not obstruct acquisition and/or expression of information and so inhibit intellectual/mental development, are essential to everything we do. It is therefore critically important for learning in all other subject areas that any individual's ability to read and convey information in the written form of the language is as good as it can possibly be.

Especially in the context of academic development, significant difficulties and underperformance in reading and writing often generate emotional and social difficulties—and sometimes behavioural difficulties too.

## Implications for assessment

The chain of causation stretching back from poor phonological awareness and consequent ability to apply the related skills and knowledge to word identification, through poor phonological representation to poorly developed precursor skills—and perhaps beyond—taken as the defining characteristics, means that the assessment for dyslexia must focus on these. The assessment must show that there is poor phonological skills application and, by implication, poor phonological awareness, further implying poor phonological representation.

It is not possible to measure/assess the struggle to develop appropriate levels of fluency in the use of the written language in a one-off assessment, but there should be evidence of that and of adequate opportunity to learn these in the history of the assessed (that history, if available in the detail really required, may even then not show that the opportunity was taken by the learner).

The discrepancy between IQ and reading performance will show only that the problem is specific and, since it is only a once-off measurement, it cannot show a history of struggle to learn. One of the critical measures in all this will be word identification—inferred from word recognition test performance. Phonological skills/awareness may also be inferred to some extent from such tests.

## Implications for remediation

Insofar as the distinction between SRR and GRR learners is at all useful, it suggests that GRR learners also need help in general intellectual development. Both groups need help in remedying their difficulties in word identification and spelling skills.

## The place of IQ in reading and spelling performance

For many years the major way—still practised by some—of identifying dyslexia was by measurement of the discrepancy between performance on reading or spelling tests and in a test of IQ—usually one of the Weschler intelligence scales. Setting aside for the moment the contentious issues surrounding the nature of IQ and its measurement, and the actual nature and information produced by the Weschler tests, this means of identifying developmental dyslexia is based on the proposition that reading ability should somehow be at the same level as IQ of this type. This is because there is a positive correlation between the two. However, this proposition has, over the last fifteen years, been shown to be untenable for several reasons.

Firstly, although there is a positive correlation between the two, this does not indicate cause. It indicates only that there is a sharing of variance—or cause. It is more than likely that the cause is a third entity and, if one of these **does** cause the other, it's more likely that reading causes 'intelligence' by increasing the information stored. Secondly, most recent research shows that the correlation between the two is in the order of only about 9 per cent, that is, 91 per cent of the variance is **not** shared! In children, there is, in fact, a bigger correlation beween IQ and shoe size, the reason being that as one gets older, one's feet increase in size and (quite separately of course) one acquires more information and so do better on IQ tests! No one would argue cause from **this** correlation!

Thirdly, recent research also shows that difference in IQ did not indicate difference in struggle to learn the skills of reading and writing, nor difference in their rate of improvement between groups of very young learners, one of which had higher IQ than the other. That said, the difference between the two sets of scores can provide **some** useful information. It can indicate whether the difficulty in learning is general or specific to developing fluency in the skills of reading and communicating in writing. So, what is the point of measuring IQ in trying to identify dyslexia or classify individuals as dyslexic? And, given the other propositions that people with 'inadequate IQ' (whatever that turns out to be) can't possibly be dyslexic, how 'intelligent' do you have to be to successfully learn to read?

The answer to the first question is that the battery of tests, of which, for example, the Weschler scales are composed, includes assessment of abilities such as oral vocabulary and verbal reasoning, which **are** relevant to the development of the ability to read and write—so the information obtained from these can be helpful. The answer to the second question is more complex and will be addressed in detail after more detailed consideration of the information produced by 'IQ' tests such as Weschler's.

*General intellectual functioning* (as assessed by tests such as the Weschler intelligence scales): Assessment of major functions of the brain which are involved in intellectual activities, measured and grouped together to give an estimate of the intellectual mental functioning of the brain as a whole. Each area or activity is measured separately and the results expressed in the form of a scale score for that activity. These results are then grouped into two main groupings: those in which intellectual functioning is tested through the medium of words—verbally mediated activities—and those which are tested through the medium of visual presentation and physical response—i.e. as in arranging things in the manner of a jigsaw. The results of these groupings are expressed as an IQ score and these two Verbal Scale and Non-Verbal or Performance Scale scores are then combined into a total or Full Scale score, also expressed as an IQ score.

*IQ (Intelligence Quotient):* This figure is the result of a division operation—a quotient—in this case the 'mental age' (see below) of a person divided by their chronological (actual) age. However, since dividing the average ten year old's mental age of ten by their chronological age of ten would give an IQ of one, this figure is **arbitrarily** multiplied by 100 to give an IQ of 100. In addition, because the 'mental age' score changes with normal day-to-day changes in the performance of all individuals on such tasks, a correction figure, called the Standard Error of Measurement, which takes account of the variation in test performance, as well as the imperfections in all mental tests, is applied; so the notional average IQ of 100 is actually 100 plus or minus 4–5. In addition, because of variability in performance in mental tests of the groups tested, the actual average score of the average person lies within the range of 100 plus or minus 15; i.e. the IQ scores in the range 85 to 115 are **all** taken as being average. This is called the standard deviation.

*Intelligence:* Unfortunately there are many definitions of intelligence and the only one accepted by **all** workers in the field is 'that which intelligence tests measure'. Tests of general intellectual function measure only some aspects of a wide range of abilities of which the human brain is capable. For example, the Weschler tests of intelligence measure a range of functions; e.g. oral vocabulary, mental arithmetic and part of the capacity for reasoning using words, as well as the ability to reason using clues in drawings, and the ability to perceive relationships between the bits of a drawing of a common object which has been cut into pieces and put them together to make the whole picture without the aid of a complete picture of the object, such as is provided in jigsaw puzzles.

Other definitions, and tests, of intelligence are of verbal and/or numerical and/or non-verbal reasoning and are usually tests in which there is thought to be only one correct answer on which the person tested converges by a process of logical reasoning. For this reason they are known in the psychology profession as convergent reasoning tests.

A third definition of intelligence is that of non-verbal reasoning only, which uses the ability to converge on the right answer in puzzles not involving words. These puzzles are composed of sets of drawings or diagrams which are related to each other in some way. Identifying the way in which they are related to each other will lead the person tested to the 'right' answer.

It is important to note that **all** of these different tests, as well as others, produce a final score expressed as IQ—even though their content is not the same. This is a particularly important issue when the IQ score is used as a benchmark against which performances in other mental functions such as reading are considered. For example, difficulty in reading, writing and spelling may be considered in the context of other intellectual functions, such as oral vocabulary and verbally-mediated reasoning which support them. If, for example, performance in reading accuracy is much lower than performances in most, if not all, other intellectual function generally, the underfunctioning or underachievement is said to be **specific**. As seen from the descriptions above, this can be demonstrated by comparing the reading test score to that obtained from the relevant parts of the Weschler tests, for example, but not to others, such as tests of diagrammatic reasoning, because these measure unrelated specific functions.

A working definition of intelligence as commonly understood might be:

> *the ability to understand the nature of a problem or task (or question) presented and organise and produce the most appropriate and relevant response to that "problem".*

It may be seen that this ability depends on a range of skills and knowledge which must be learned, usually by experience, often informally and not necessarily by deliberate or formal teaching. Humans have the fewest number of pre-programmed responses.

*Mental age:* This is an estimate of mental ability, usually a range of scholastic type intellectual activities, which is derived by subjecting a large number of people to tests of these activities in order to obtain an average score for persons of their age which then serves as a 'norm' or benchmark against which the scores of individuals can be compared.

For example, if all ten year olds in the UK are measured for their performance in reading accuracy, mental arithmetic, oral vocabulary, general knowledge, knowledge of the rules of social behaviour, reading comprehension and ability to solve diagrammatic puzzles, and the total scores of all of them are grouped together, this would give the average score of the average ten year old in these functions. In practice, this is not actually possible so the 'norm' is created on a **relatively small sample** of ten year olds.

Therefore, the 'mental age' of the 'average' ten year old in the UK calculated in this way would be used as a basis of comparison—a benchmark—for other ten year olds whose intellectual functioning is subsequently assessed individually.

It should be noted that all of these mental functions are **learned**—albeit on a variable base of biological development—and are therefore subject to many factors, for example time spent in school, motivation to learn scholastic activities, freedom from physical or emotional obstructions to learning—all things which are involved in learning and performance.

It is now time to turn to consideration of how much 'intelligence' (and of what kind) is needed to successfully learn to read and write.

## Reading, intelligence and dyslexia

One of the criteria cited in the 'diagnosis' of developmental dyslexia is that of adequate intelligence. It is said that possession of at least 'adequate' intelligence allows the rejection of the possibility that 'inadequate intelligence' is the cause of the poor reading performance and/or errors made. This notion is then extended to become the basis of the idea that the discrepancy between intelligence and reading ability defines developmental dyslexia. But is it? And how much intelligence do you need to be able to read—or to be able to learn to read?

### Reading for meaning

Since the purpose in reading is to acquire information, the information made available in the form of the written word will be meaningful only if there is at least some pre-existing information about that topic already possessed by the reader. This is likely to be in the form of concepts stored in secondary memory and that is one form of intelligence. The more knowledge the reader has, the more meaningful the incoming information will be and, if it is new information, concepts will be expanded, further interlinking of concepts should also occur and so learning has taken place. This process is enhanced by good organisation of the incoming information, considering its relevance in as many ways and to as many existing concepts as possible. This is another form of intelligence.

Reading in this sense therefore enables the development of intelligence, at least of this type, by providing access to information but it is clearly necessary for the reader to possess a minimum of information on the topic they are reading about, if it is to make sense to them. So, reading in its essential form requires a modicum of some aspects of intelligence but reading itself also enhances these and probably other aspects of intelligence because it is a means of acquiring information. This process may be seen as an upward spiral.

## Reading accuracy (word recognition)

A different kind of reading, in the sense of word recognition, is seen in most single word reading tests. The ability to recognise words is, of course, a necessary part of the process which conveys information from the page to the brain and so is a sub- or enabling skill within the reading process generally. In order to recognise a word, it is necessary for the concept surrounding the information contained by any given word, as well as the word-form itself, to be already in the memory of the reader in the form of either the visual version or at least the sound version of the word. This is yet another aspect of intelligence. Viewing words for which there is no pre-existing concept will result in non-recognition of the word. If the verbal 'label' (that is visual or aural word-form) of that concept is also already possessed, then the two are matched and recognition takes place. If only the sound version of the verbal label already exists, the word read may be recognised if the visual form is re-coded into the sound version by using the appropriate sub-skills of reading/word identification to produce the usual sound of the word which should then be recognised.

It sometime happens that the word identification skills may be appropriately and accurately applied but the result is a word-sound which is not the one normally used for the concept. A famous example of that is the word 'colonel' which should be [kolonel] as in the original French for 'head of a column in the army', but which, in English has become distorted to [k^nl]. The intelligence required for this task includes the knowledge of the relationship between the written and spoken forms. Lack of this—or lack of knowledge of the concept or meaning—also results in the production of mispronunciations and failure to derive meaning.

It should also be clear that possession of the knowledge of how words are constructed (both acoustically and visually—phonology and its visual counterpart) and skill in application of that knowledge are yet other forms of intelligence necessary for reading in the sense of capacity for identification of words to enable their recognition and, in turn, gain access to the meaning or information they convey.

It is evident that the better the store of concepts generally, and of these in the form of spoken form of words, and the ability to manipulate ideas in verbal form, the easier it will be to read. It is therefore necessary for the reader to possess these aspects of intelligence, at least to some extent, for the development of skill in reading. But the extent to which this is necessary is debatable. A rough guide might be that at any given point on the continuum of development of skill in reading, the learner reader should possess **sufficient** of these capacities for the words which they are trying to read, and there are several adequate tests of these pieces of knowledge currently available. However, this does not justify the assertion that any individual's reading should be at the same level as their intelligence since neither causes the other.

Moreover, tests of other kinds of intelligence, for example diagrammatic or non-verbal reasoning, have little or no bearing on the processes involved in reading and spelling and therefore provide no information on these. Such capacities are not prerequisites for the development of reading and writing.

Therefore, the relevant parts of the WISC and similar tests are the verbal scale subtests of verbal reasoning (similarities), vocabulary and information—although, of these, the vocabulary test is probably the only one which gives a good measure of the intelligence actually required. Other information might be derived from other tests, for example the Slingerland and Illinois Test of Linguistic Ability (ITPA) tests, which are available to teachers as are other vocabulary and verbal reasoning tests. The only one not available to anybody is a good test of relevant knowledge.

The other subtests of the WISC and British Ability Scale (BAS) are useful in the diagnosis of dyslexia in that they may give indications of possible visual or motor problems and, in that respect, may be more relevant for the identification of dyspraxia.

Note also that **none** of the foregoing assesses **learning!** If in doubt—seek professional advice!

# Some sources of further reading

## Dyslexia

Berlin (1887) *Eine Besondere Art der Wortblindheit* (Dyslexia) Wiesbaden, Berlin

### Case reports

Bruns (1888) *Neurologisches Centralblatt*, nos 2 and 3
Nieden (1887) *Archiv fur Augenheilkunde*. Fax 2
Uhthoff (1890) *Deutsche Medizinal Zeitung*

Broadbent, Sir William (1896) Objection to Hinshelwood's use of 'wordblindness'. *Lancet* 1: 18

Bryant P, Bradley L (1986) *Children's Reading Problems*. Blackwell, Oxford

Chalfant JC, Scheffelin MA (1969) *Central Processing Dysfunctions in Children—A Review of Research NINDS Monograph No 9*. US Department of Health, Education and Welfare, Washington, DC

Chasty HT (1979) Towards an understanding of dyslexia. *Dyslexia Rev* 2(2)

Coltheart M (1976) *Deep Dyslexia*. Routledge and Keegan Paul, London

Crystal D, ed (1987) *Child Language, Learning and Linguistics*. Edward Arnold, London: Ch 2 and Ch 3

Developmental Nuerology and Learning Disorders (1982) *Dyslexia Review* 5(1)

Ellis A (1993) Reading, Writing and Dyslexia, 2nd edn

Ellis A (1984) Reading, Writing and Dyslexia

Ellis A, Young A (2000) *Human Cognitive Neuropsychology*, 2nd edn. Psychology Press, Hove

Frith U (1980) *Cognitive Processes in Spelling.* Academic Press, Philadelphia

Geschwind N (1972) Language and the brain. *Scientific American* **April**: 76

Goswami U (2002) *How to Beat Dyslexia* (the rhythm of the English language) Broadbent Memorial Lecture to the Annual Conference of the BPsS

Goswami U (1994) Reading by analogy theoretical and practical perspectives. In: Hulme C, Snowling M, eds. *Reading Development and Dyslexia.* Whurr Publishing, London

Gregory R, ed (1987) *The Oxford Companion to the Mind.* Oxford University Press, Oxford

Hinshelwood J (1917) *Congenital Word Blindness.* HK Lewis

Hinshelwood J (1896) A case of dyslexia—a peculiar form of word blindness. *Lancet* **2**: 1431–53

Hinshelwood J (1895) Word blindness and visual memory. *Lancet* **1**: 1564

Hinshelwood J (1896) Reply to Broadbent. *Lancet* **1**: 196

Jaeger-Adams M (1994) Learning to read: modelling the reader versus modelling the learner. In: Hulme C, Snowling M, eds. *Reading Development and Dyslexia.* Whurr Publishing, London

Kennedy A *The Psychology of Reading.*

Kerr J (1896) School hygiene in its mental, moral and physical aspects. *J Roy Statist Soc* **60**: 613–80

Long M (2001) *Dyslexia—what it is and what we should do about it*: www.psych-ed.org/Topics/Dyslexia.htm

McGuinness D (1998) *Why Children Can't Read and What we Can Do About It.* Penguin, Harmondsworth

Pavlidis, Miles (1981) *Dyslexia Research and Its Application to Education.*

Pirrozolo FK (1979) *The Neuropsychology of Developmental Reading Disorders.* Praeger, Westport, CT

Pringle Morgan W (1896) A case of congenital word blindness. *Br Med J* **2**: 1378

Pumfrey P, Reason R (1991) *Specific Learning Difficulties* (Dyslexia).

Some sources of further reading

Rosner J (1993) *Helping Children Overcome Learning Difficulties*, 2nd edn. Walker & Co, New York; Beaverbooks, Canada

Rutter M, Yule W (1975) The concept of specific reading retardation. *J Child Psychol Psychiatry* **16**: 181–97

Seymour PHK, Porpodas CD (1980) Lexical and non-lexical processing of spelling in developmental dyslexia. In: Frith U, ed. *Cognitive Processing in Reading and Spelling*. Academic Press, London

Smith F (1978) *Reading*. Cambridge University Press, Cambridge

Snowling MJ (2000) *Dyslexia* 2nd edn.

Snowling MJ, ed (1986) *Children's Written Language Difficulties*.

Snowling MJ (1986) *Developmental Dyslexia—A Cognitive Approach*.

Snowling MJ (1980) Dyslexia—where is the deficit? *Dyslexia Rev* **3**(1):

Stein JF, Fowler S (1985) Effect of monocular occlusion on visuomotor perception and reading in dyslexic children. *Lancet* **2**(8446): 69–73

Vernon MD (1977) Deficiencies in dyslexics. *Dyslexia Rev* summer (17):

## Psychology

Gregory R, ed (1987) *The Oxford Companion to the Mind*. Oxford University Press, Oxford

Hildegard, Atkinson (1993) *Psychology. Introduction to Psychology*, 11th edn. Harcourt Brace, Fortworth: ch 2

Sluckin L, *et al* (1970) *Introducing psychology: an experimental approach*. In: Wright DS, Taylor A, Reason JT, eds. Penguin, Harmondsworth

## Brain structure and function

(1982) Developmental neurology and learning disorders. *Dyslexia Rev* **5**(1):

Berlin (1981; revised 1985) *Left Brain, Right Brain*. Springer and Deutsch ; (revised) 1985 WH Freeman & Co, New York

Chalfant JC, Scheffelin MA (1969) *Central Processing Dysfunctions in Children—A Review of Research*, NINDS Monograph No 9. US Department of Health, Education and Welfare, Washington, DC

Development neurology and learning disorders (1982) *Dyslexia Rev* 5(1)

Dimond, Beaumont (1983) *Hemispherical Function in the Human Brain.*

Geschwind N (1972) Language and the brain. *Scientific American* April: 76

Kimura D (1961) *Cerebral Dominance in the Disabled Reader.* ?publisher/place?

Kinsbourne M, Warrington EK (1963) Developmental factors in reading and writing backwardness. *Br J Psychol* 54: 145–56

Luria AR (1973) *The Working Brain.* Penguin, Hardmondsworth: *et seq*

Maguire, *et al* (2000) Navigation-related structural change in the hippocampi of taxi drivers. *Proc Nat Acad Sci* 97(8): 4378–403

Pirozzolo FJ (1979) *The Neuropsychology of Developmental Reading Disorders.* Praeger, Connecticut

Rasmussen, Milner (1975) *Clinical and Surgical Studies of Cerebral Speech Areas.*

Saffran E (1982) Neurological approaches to the study of language. Br J Psychiatry?/Psychology? ?vol no?(?issue no?): ?page nos?

Sandstrom ?initial? (?year?) *From Childhood to Adolescence.* ?publisher/place?

Wolpert L (1991) *The Triumph of the Embryo.* Oxford University Press, Oxford

## Language development and use

Crystal D (1987) *Child Language, Learning and Linguistics.* Edward Arnold, London: Ch 2; Ch 3

Crystal D (1987) *The Cambridge Encyclopaedia of Language.* Cambridge University Press, Cambridge

# Some sources of further reading

de Villiers PA, de Villiers JG(1979)In: Bruner, ed. *'DaDa' Early Language*. Fontana Books, Harmondsworth

Goswami U (1994) Reading by analogy: theoretical and practical perspectives. In: Hulme C, Snowling MJ, eds. *Reading Development and Dyslexia*. Whurr Publishing, London

Harley T (2001) The Psychology of Language. The Psychology Press, Taylor and Francis, London

Jaeger-Adams M (1994) Modelling the reader versus modelling the learner. In: Hulme C, Snowling MJ, eds. *Reading Development and Dyslexia*. Whurr Publishing, London

Potter S (1971) *Our Language*. Penguin, Harmondsworth

Potter S (1957) Modern Linguistics. Andre Deutsch

Skinner BF (1957) *Verbal Behavior*. Appleton Century Crofts, New York

Skinner BF (1953) *Verbal Learning*. Appleton Century Crofts, New York

## Learning

Borger R, Seaborne AEM (1966) *The Psychology of Learning*. Pelican, Harmondsworth

Gagne RM (1964) *The Conditions of Learning*. Holt, Rinehart & Winston, Austin, TX

Holt J (1972) *How Children Fail*. Pitman Publishing, Bristol

Rosner J (1979) *Helping Children Overcome Learning Difficulties*. Walker & Co, New York; Beaverbooks, Canada

Rutter M, Yule W (1975) The concept of specific reading retardation. *J Child Psychol Psychiatry* 16: 181–97

Skinner BF (1957) *Verbal Behavior*. Appleton Century Crofts, New York

## Perception

Barber P, Legge D (1976) Perception and information. In: *Essential Psychology*. Methuen, London

Barber P, Legge D (1976) Information and skill. In: *Essential Psychology*. Methuen, London

Knight R, Knight M (1964) *A Modern Introduction to Psychology*. University Tutorial Press, London

Moray N (1969) Attention Selective Processes in Vision and Hearing. Hutchinson Educational Books, Random House, New York

Rosner J (1979) *Helping Children Overcome Learning Difficulties*. Walker & Co, New York; Beaverbooks, Canada

## Memory

Baddeley A (1986) *Working Memory*. Oxford University Press, Oxford

Baddeley A (1982) *Memory—A User's Guide*. Avery Penguin Putnam, Harmondsworth

Baddeley A, Hitch GJ (1974) Working memory. In: Bower G ed. *Recent Advances in Learning and Motivation*, Vol VIII. Academic Press, New York

*Experiments in STM Using Digits*. Also Post Office Telecomms experiments in misdialling.

Gregg V (1975) *Human Memory*. Methuen Paperback Series on Essential Psychology. Methuen, London

Postman L, Keppel G, eds (1969) *Verbal Learning and Memory Reading*. Penguin, Harmondsworth

Rosner J (1979) *Helping Children Overcome Learning Difficulties*. Walker & Co, New York; Beaverbooks, Canada

## Reading, spelling and writing

Bryant P, Bradley L (1986) *Children's Reading Problems*. Blackwell, Oxford

Craigie, Sir William (1937) *Spelling*. SPE Tract 93, London

Goswami U, Bryant P (1999) Phonological skills and learning to read. In: Goswami U, Bryant P, eds. *Essays in Developmental Psychology*. Psychology Press, Hove

Kennedy A (1984) *The Psychology of Reading*. Methuen, London

Rosner J (1979) *Helping Children Overcome Learning Difficulties.* Walker & Co, New York; Beaverbooks, Canada

Schonell F (1961) *The Psychology and Teaching of Reading.* Oliver and Boyd, Edinburgh

Smith F (1978) *Reading.* Cambridge University Press, Cambridge

## Some useful journal/newspaper articles, etc

Papers in the *British Journal of Psychology,*
*British Journal of Educational Psychology*
*British Journal Of Developmental Psychology*—published quarterly by the British Psychological Society.

Also papers in specialist journals such as *Brain* and *Literacy Today*.

Other, usually journalistic and often inaccurate, reports appear in the newspapers from time to time. Examples of these are:

Spelling. *Guardian Education* Insert 20 October 1992

Spoken vs Written Language Usage. *Independent on Sunday* 7 February 1993

Report on success of Clay Reading Recovery System in *Surrey Daily Mail* February 1993

# Glossary of terms used

*Acquisition (in memory):* the acquiring of information—normally into long-term storage—a very complex operation which results in learning if the information acquired adds to or expands related information already in store, as for example in reading.

Difficulty in acquisition, including retention and/or combining with existing stores, is most frequently the cause of 'forgetting'—difficulty in recall or retrieval—since the information was never stored in the first place and cannot therefore be 'recalled'. This can happen in reading and spelling.

*Communication in writing or in written form:* the transmission of information (in the sense used in the study of brain processes) in the form of the written language (which, in English, uses arbitrary symbols), normally to a receiver in another time or place—so precluding the use of the spoken form. This includes things such as the knowledge of the effects of punctuation and the skilled use of that, as well as the production of the visual form of words, and is distinct from 'writing' in the literal sense of the physical/motor activity of forming or drawing letter and word-shapes.

*General intellectual functioning:* (as assessed by tests such as the Weschler intelligence scales). Assessment of major functions of the brain which are involved in intellectual activities, measured and grouped together to give an estimate of the intellectual mental functioning of the brain as a whole. Each area or activity is measured separately and the results expressed in the form of a scale score for that activity. These results are then grouped into two main groupings: those in which intellectual functioning is tested through the medium of words—verbally mediated activities—and those which are tested through the medium of visual presentation and physical response—such as in arranging things in the manner of a jigsaw. The results of these groupings are expressed as an 'IQ' score and these two Verbal Scale and Non-Verbal or Performance Scale scores are then combined into a total or Full Scale score, also expressed as an 'IQ' score.

*Intelligence:* Unfortunately there are many definitions of intelligence and the only one accepted by **all** workers in the field is 'that which intelligence tests measure'. Tests of general intellectual function measure some aspects of a wide range of abilities of which the human brain is capable. For example, the Weschler tests of intelligence measure a range of functions like oral vocabulary, mental arithmetic and part of the capacity for reasoning using words, as well as the ability to reason using clues in drawings and the ability to perceive relationships between the bits of a drawing of a common object which has been cut into pieces and put together to make the whole picture without the aid of a complete picture of the object, such as is provided in jigsaw puzzles.

Other definitions, and tests, of intelligence are of verbal and/or numerical and/or non-verbal reasoning and are usually tests in which there is thought to be only one correct answer on which the person tested converges by a process of logical reasoning. For this reason they are known in the psychology profession as convergent reasoning tests.

A third definition of intelligence is that of non-verbal reasoning only, which is the ability to converge on the right answer in puzzles not involving words. These puzzles are composed of sets of drawings or diagrams that are related to each other in some way. Identifying the way in which they are related to each other will lead the person tested to the 'right' answer.

It is important to note that **all** of these different tests as well as others produce a final score expressed as IQ—even though their content is not the same. This is a particularly important issue when the IQ score is used as a baseline against which performances in other mental functions, such as reading, are considered. For example, difficulty in reading, writing and spelling may be considered in the context of other intellectual functions, such as oral vocabulary and verbally-mediated reasoning, which support them. If performance in reading accuracy is much lower than performances in most, if not all, other intellectual functions generally, the underfunctioning or underachievement is said to be **specific**. As can be seen from the descriptions above, this can be demonstrated by comparing the reading test score to that obtained from the relevant parts of the Weschler tests, for example, but not to tests of diagrammatic reasoning, for instance, because these measure unrelated specific functions.

A working definition of intelligence as commonly understood might be:
*'the ability to understand the nature of a problem or task (or question) presented and organise and produce the most appropriate and relevant response to that "problem".'*

It may be seen that this ability depends on a range of skills and knowledge which must be learned, usually by experience, often informally and not necessarily by deliberate or formal teaching. Humans have the fewest number of pre-programmed responses.

*IQ (Intelligence Quotient):* This figure is the result of a division operation—a quotient—in this case the 'mental age' (see below) of a person divided by their chronological (actual) age. However, since dividing the average ten year old's mental age of ten by their chronological age of ten would give an IQ of one, this figure is **arbitrarily** multiplied by 100 to give an IQ of 100. In addition, because the 'mental age' score changes with normal day-to-day changes in the performance of all individuals on such tasks, a correction figure, called the Standard Error of Measurement, which takes account of the variation in test performance as well as the imperfections in all mental tests, is applied, so the notional average IQ of 100 is actually 100 plus or minus 4–5. In addition to that, also because of variability in performance in mental tests of groups tested, the actual average score of the average person lies within the range of 100 plus or minus 15. That is, the IQ scores in the range 85 to 115 are all taken as being average. This is called the standard deviation.

*Learning:* the change/increase in the 'information' possessed and/or the behaviour/response repertoire available (the term 'information' is used here to mean **any** piece of knowledge in **any** of the forms used by the senses **or** in verbal [word] form and not in its usual general sense).

*Learning difficulty:* inordinate difficulty in learning or achieving a particular learning target. This may have a number of distinct possible causes which may also act in concert. Some of these potential causes, assuming adequate motivation and commitment, are: inappropriate learning targets and/or inappropriate learning methods and/or inappropriate learning strategies (all of these may be either teacher or self-determined—sometimes wilfully); inappropriate learning skills base and/or inadequate information base. These may bring about an apparent 'inability' to learn but only insofar as they are allowed to persist.

Strictly speaking, identification of a **learning** difficulty requires two or more measurements of performance of the function or ability, preferably interspersed with periods of learning or development of the ability or knowledge in question, to determine whether or not learning is taking place (see **Learning** above).

A single measurement of performance is just that—**performance at the time tested.**

*Long-term memory:* the permanent storage of information in the brain. Popularly misunderstood and misused to mean memory of events which took place a long time ago. Also called permanent or secondary memory.

*Memory:* the storage of information—initially in the form of the senses through which it was acquired, but ultimately in the form of very complex and changeable inter-related concepts. This may be seen if one hears something familiar and gets a simultaneous mental image of an occurrence or event in which that sound was a strong feature, even though no visual image is present.

*Mental age:* this is an estimate of mental ability, usually a range of scholastic type intellectual activities, which is derived by subjecting a large number of people to tests of these activities in order to obtain an average score for persons of their age which then serves as a 'norm' or 'benchmark' against which the scores of individuals can be compared. For example, if all ten year olds in the UK are measured for their performance in reading accuracy, mental arithmetic, oral vocabulary, general knowledge, knowledge of the rules of social behaviour, reading comprehension and ability to solve diagrammatic puzzles, and the total scores of all of them are grouped together, this would give the average score of the average ten year old in these functions. In practice, this is not actually possible so the 'norm' is created on a **sample** of ten yearolds.

Therefore, the 'mental age' of the 'average' ten year old in the UK calculated in this way would be used as a basis of comparison—a 'benchmark'—for other ten year olds whose intellectual functioning is subsequently assessed individually.

It should be noted that all of these mental functions are learned—albeit on a variable base of biological development—and therefore subject to the many factors, such as time spent in school, motivation to learn scholastic activities, freedom from physical or emotional obstructions to learning—which are involved in learning and performance.

*Motor:* (as in motor control and co-ordination)—the activity in specific areas of the brain which initiates and controls movement of any part of the body.

*Perception:* the ability to comprehend or understand the 'meaning'—in this context of something heard or seen. For example, the actual image of any shape falling on the retina of the eye is back to front and upside down (because the lens of the eye is curved) but the brain corrects for this and 'perceives' it the right way up and the right way round.

In addition, if a baseball cap is drawn looking at it from the left side and the peak to the left, and the viewers knows that that is what it is supposed to be, no matter how it is turned around, it always represents—or 'means'—a baseball cap. This is called perceptual constancy. If, however, the very same shape, when it is placed in one way, or orientation, is agreed by everyone to be a 'p' and the same shape in another orientation agreed to be a 'b', the reader must learn—arbitrarily since these is no 'natural' logic in this—that the orientation of the shape determines its meaning, as in the case of the 'baseball cap' becoming 'p' or 'b' or 'd' or 'q'.

*Phonological:* to do with the sounds with which words are made up—their sound structures. Phonology is the study of these structures and the effects they have on the meaning they convey.

*Phonological awareness:* the awareness of the way words are made up of sound structures—sometimes of single letters and sometimes of part words (syllables or morphemes), such as common endings like '-ing'. This knowledge is used as the basis of the skill of identifying the sounds within a word being read and saying them aloud so that the word, hopefully a known word in the individual's oral vocabulary, will be recognised. This process is also known as the technique of 'Phonics'.

*Phonetics:* the arrangement or description of the 44 basic speech sounds (phones) used in the English language in accordance with the position in the mouth where they are made. This is normally shown in a diagram of these positions by those who study phonology.

*Phoneme:* this term is normally and inaccurately used to mean the sound that a letter makes as if the letter represented only one sound. Since there are only 26 letters in the English language and at least 44 separate sounds, this is not possible.

Phonemics actually describe the relationships of the individual phones and the meaning they carry when used in specific words in the spoken language—especially in regional or dialect variations. For example, in the word 'but', the dialect of the south of England pronounces the 'u' as [uh] but in the north of England the sound made is almost [oo] as in 'boot', **yet the meaning remains the same.** Because of that, the sounds made are said to be different allophones or variants of the same phoneme—even though the **phones** are different. Where the change in sound causes a change in meaning (as it would in this case if the sounds were made **only** by a southern speaker in 'but' and 'boot', then the [uh] and the [oo] are treated as **different** phonemes. In some southern dialects, [f] and [th] and sometimes [v] are very frequently allophones of the phoneme 'f'.

A phoneme is therefore the **range** of phones or sounds which can be used within all of any word's regional variations **without changing its meaning**. This is important for learning to read and spell in dialects other than that of southern England.

## *Reading:*

1   The ability or skills to acquire or extract information from written or printed text (at least in this context. *Reading Comprehension.* There are other, broader, equally valid meanings, such as reading a map or reading the weather signs and even reading a person's attitudes or intentions from the expression on their face).

   The assessment of reading ability actually falls into three categories and the tests reflect these but are more often, wrongly, used interchangeably.

   The fundamental aspect of reading is that of reading comprehension. It is sometimes forgotten that there are all kinds of phenomena within this function which aid its performance—for example, the redundancy of the text, the adequacy of concept store (store of 'knowledge' of/familiarity with the subject matter) of the reader for the task and the very complex mental activity of perception of meaning.

2   The ability to recognise written or printed words. *Word Recognition.* Word recognition is also known as reading 'accuracy'. The results may show, by chance, only some of the words known by the individual but give an estimate of the extent and nature of the words which they immediately recognise. The set of words which any individual can be expected to recognise is actually specific to that individual and depends on many things, for example their experience of their environment for the formation of knowledge of the world around them and especially the words used to describe it and their experience of the words in print. There should be some relationship, but not an exact one, between their word recognition vocabulary and their oral vocabulary.

3   *Word Identification* (also known as word attack): the ability to **identify** written or printed words which are not immediately

recognised. This is based on adequate awareness of the phonology—the sound structure—of the spoken language and usually achieved by application of word identification skills of analysis of a word into syllables, morphemes (part-word) or single sounds (phonemes), then synthesis or 'blending' of these parts into whole words which may then be recognised from their whole word sounds. For some words, the use of additional knowledge and skills is also necessary.

Assessment is made on the individual's performance in application of phonological analysis, knowledge of letter/sound relationships—particularly of groups of letters—and then synthesising or 'blending' these discrete sounds into a unified pattern. The purpose—of which the user must be made aware—of these techniques is to hear and possibly recognise an oral or sound version of a word which is already known to them (already in their oral vocabulary). If the individual does not already possess it in memory in sound form, the pattern produced by analysis and blending in this manner may not be recognised. It is also possible that the correct operation of word identification skills will not produce the usual, and therefore recognisable, sound-form of the word, as for example if the child correctly segments 'canary' into 'can' and 'arry' which when put together then produces 'cannery', a very different word—and a very common mistake.

*Recall (or retrieval) (in memory):* the searching for and bringing into play (for example in constructing the answer to a question) of information stored in permanent memory.

*Remembering:* a popular but imprecise and often inaccurate phrase used to describe one or more of the activities and functions actually operational in memory. It is most often used to mean the act of recall but also frequently of acquisition and storage.

*Retention (in memory):* the holding of information—usually, in the context of reading or spelling—for a short period while it is being 'worked on' in 'working memory'.

*Self-managed learning:* the design and implementation of a programme of learning for oneself. Also used to mean implementation of a learning programme devised by someone else.

*Semantic:* relating to meaning. Most things are thought to be stored in memory in accordance with their 'meaningfulness' for the person whose memories they are.

*Short-term memory:* the ability to retain information of whatever kind for very short duration. Popularly misunderstood and misused to mean memory of recent events.

*Specific learning difficulty:* in the context of reading difficulty, an apparent difficulty only in developing the skills of reading and/or communicating in writing (including spelling). This is seldom actually established. What is normally measured is performance and so what is exposed is specific **performance** difficulty. Specific **learning** difficulty is assumed or inferred from a significant discrepancy between performances in the tasks of an intelligence test, such as the WISC, and in reading or spelling tests or **persistent** difficulty.

The inference is made that, since the individual has evidently developed 'general intelligence' to a 'normal' extent, but their ability to read or write has apparently not developed to anything like the same extent, they must have a learning difficulty (which in this context is often—wrongly—assumed to be an **inability** to learn) which is specific to these functions. This is questionable. The actual **causes** of the difficulty are a different issue.

*Spelling:* the ability to produce the 'written' form of words. This can either be in the context of spontaneous intent to communicate information in the 'written' form of the language or in response to specific requests to produce specific words presented in a list of spoken words—usually out of their normal context—in the form of 'dictation'.

The 'correct' form or 'spelling' of words in the English language is now often arbitrary and there are two major routes or strategies for the production of words—spelling. These are known technically as 'addressed spelling' and 'assembled spelling'.

**Addressed spelling** is the form used by skilled spellers until they encounter a word which is not visually familiar to them, at which point they will usually and properly switch to the use of the complementary skill of assembled spelling.

In addressed spelling, the speller knows (has a complete and accurate visual image in permanent memory of) the visual form of the word they are spelling and 'addresses' or accesses that memory store directly when the need arises to write it down. The visual image in memory is then drawn or 'written' (perhaps typed).

**Assembled spelling** is the conversion of the **sound** version of the word stored in permanent memory, bit by bit, into the letters which represent these sounds. During this process, the sound version of the word is apparently held temporarily in 'working' memory (see below).

In assembled spelling, the speller is primarily working on sounds—usually because their 'memory' of the visual form of the word in question is either absent or incomplete—and depending on a range of sub-skills to help them convert these sounds into letter and word form, frequently resulting in 'phonic' or 'phonetic' spelling where the word is not the 'correct' visual version but, if read aloud, produces the 'correct' original sound.

It also appears that less skilled spellers—those who do not have a large store of the relevant visual images of words—may often use a combination of conversion of the sounds within words and also some half-remembered or poor visual representations of the words, and this can be mutually obstructive when attempts to use the poor visual images interfere with the smooth operation of conversion of the sound form of the word, bit by bit, into the 'written' form.

Unfortunately, in the English language, there is often no fixed relationship even between the 26 letters and the 44 single sounds they are used to represent, although there are many commonly occurring words and part words.

For this reason, assembled spelling is, by its very nature, subject to probability—the likelihood that in **this** word the sounds are represented by **these** letters—perhaps on the basis of use in a similar word which is familiar to the speller. It may also require the use of other, complementary techniques. For example, if one didn't know the word, using 'phonics' only might result in the less common word for the branch of a tree—'bough'—being spelled 'bow' because it sounds like the more common word 'how'. Similarly, the 'u' and 'i' letters produce quite different sounds in the words 'fruit', 'build' and 'ruin'. The only real answer to the problem of spelling unfamiliar words is to know what they look like and that means acquiring and retaining their visual image—usually during the course of reading.

*Substructures:* (Visual or phonological) the part-words within a word which make up that word and into which the word is decomposed, destructured or analysed during the process of identifying it in order to recognise and obtain its meaning. This can be done either in the word's visual parts or its sound parts. For example, the substructures of the word 'downstairs' are 'down' and 'stairs'—words in their own right which are more familiar to most people. 'Blending' them together, usually by **saying** them one after the other, should lead to the recognition of the whole word, 'downstairs'. Similarly, the substructures of 'systematic' can be 'sys' – 'tem' – 'a' – 'tic', but the individual reader might prefer 'system – atic' or 'syst – e – matic'. Whatever works for the individual is 'right'.

*Syntactic:* the word order structure in language. In the English language, the order of the words in a sentence determines or refines the ultimate meaning for the listener or reader.

*Teaching:* the provision of instruction or of the opportunity to learn; the design and implementation of a programme of learning for another.

*Tracking:* (also called scanning) in this context, the movement of the eyes across text when reading. In the English language, the movement is left to right. This activity is apparently simple but visually and mentally complex, because it appears that skilled readers do not process every aspect of the visual presentation (the words), which would be too laborious, but instead take note of only those parts of a word which distinguish it from all other words. These are known as the critical visual features for reading.

In order to do this, the skilled reader must somehow learn which are the critical visual features and therefore must learn how to look and what to look for.

*Trauma:* any experience which is of extraordinarily high emotion or state of nervous activity for the person experiencing it. A shock-like experience, such as an accident or problems surrounding birth.

*Verbal:* this means pertaining to words. It is used loosely to mean the oral or spoken version of words as distinct from the written version. In psychology and psycholinguistics, the distinction is made, of necessity, between oral/verbal and written/verbal forms and this distinction should be maintained in the study of dyslexia.

*Visual function:* in this context, those aspects of vision which are involved in reading and communicating in the written form of the language. These will include: control of the muscles which direct the eyes, the ability to follow lines of print (tracking), the ability to see 'depth' or in 'three dimensions' (convergence) and the ability to focus accurately at fixed far and near points, as well as the ability to discriminate and make sense of 'pictorial' information. To do this, one eye—the reference or 'dominant' eye—fixes on the object and the other moves to achieve convergence.

*Visual (and auditory) discrimination:* the ability to distinguish visual figures, such as letter shapes, or sounds—especially speech sounds in this context—from each other and from other similar shapes or sounds.

*(Visuo-)spatial awareness:* although this can logically also apply to sound, in this context it is most often seen in visual form. It is the ability to 'see' or perceive things in the arrangement in space in which they actually are. In cases where there is a difficulty in spatial awareness, the individual concerned—as far as we can actually tell—'sees' things closer to each other, or virtually on top of each other, or—in extreme cases—everything either to the left or to the right of their field of vision, or only half or some other part of the entire visual picture available in their field of vision. It may also take the form of difficulty in judging distance visually. It should be noted that, since any observer's knowledge of this depends on the report of the individual affected by it, it is extremely difficult to know precisely what they are, in fact, 'seeing'—especially since this is also a combination of vision and perception.

*Working memory:* a theoretical, temporary holding store of information while it is being worked on, for example in word identification in reading. The information is then either moved into permanent (long-term) memory store or discarded in a way similar to what happens to the keyboard memory in a computer when it is switched off.

# Index

## A

acquired brain damage dyslexia 22

acquired dyslexia 16, 18, 30, 34, 79, 87

  medical model of 22

assessment 8, 45–48

  for dyslexia 91, 93

  implications for 92

  of abilities 95

  of adults 51

  of major functions 95

  of reading ability 7

  one-off 93

  routine 48

## B

BPsS DECP 19, 29, 31, 33, 35–36, 41, 44, 47, 86, 89, 92

## C

communication 36, 89

  basis of 62

  in writing 9, 66

  skills 33

  spoken 77

  verbal 11, 66

  written 66

  written skills 52

concept development 58

## D

damage 15

  acquired dyslexia and 79

  brain 12–14, 18

  congenital 14

  developmental dyslexia and 30, 34

  dyslexia 45

  locus of 79

  minimal brain 82

  permanent 16

  to the brain 11

decoding 56, 58, 71, 89

developmental dyslexia 2, 11, 13, 21–23, 34–37, 42–48, 79, 83, 92

  BPsS DECP definition of 29, 32, 86

  causation in 13

  causes of 18, 33

  concept of 21

  conceptions of 19

  definition of 19, 29, 43

  definitions of 19

  described by the BPsS DECP 41

  diagnosis of 22, 98

  diagnostic system for detection of 24

  distinguishing features 30, 86

  educationally defined 20

  error forms in 16

  errors 22

  exploring further concepts 79, 81

  identifying 42, 94

  implications of the BPsS DECP definition 47

  Pavlidis and 83

  phenomenon of 15

  reading/spelling difficulties and 52

  specific learning difficulty as a sub-class 44

  specific learning difficulty as a subset of 19

  symptoms of 20

  wastebasket 89

dysfunction 1, 12–13, 79

  memory 92

## F

fMRI scanning 18, 30, 35

functional literacy 3

performance 12, 22
poor performance in 44, 47
precursor skills 18, 33
procedures and tests for assessing 49
processes involved 55
psychology of 84
retarded 30
skills 3, 26, 37, 86
specific difficulties 31
standardised tests 53
static processes 61
tests 39
reading ability
   interactions in 83
reading accuracy 99
reading and IQ
   correlation 85
reading comprehension 7, 97, 114
reading difficulties
   and the left-handed population 25
   research into 35
reading retardation
   specific 32, 85
reading skills
   development of 23
   fluency in 42
reading tactics 50
reading tests 99
reading, intelligence and dyslexia 98
redundant 56
remedial tuition 17, 32, 39, 43–44, 47, 85–86
   resistance to 33, 84

## S
secondary signalling system 55
social inclusion 4
special needs 4
specific learning difficulty 14, 19, 22, 33, 44, 82, 87, 89
   dyslexia and the notion of 15
spelling 1, 4, 7, 9, 20, 28, 36, 42–43, 52, 67, 75–77, 87–88, 91, 100
   addressed 9, 62, 69, 72, 74
   assembled 9–10, 62, 69, 73
   assessment of adults 51

development 74
difficulties in 28, 68, 96
operations in 60
phonetic 10, 74, 76
phonic 62, 72–73, 77
problems 48, 71
procedures and tests for assessing 49
processes involved in 67
rules 67, 73–74
single word test 71
skills 93
standardised tests 53
static processes in 61, 67
success in 72
tests 39, 71, 78
writing as you speak 75
written form 50
spelling performance
   place of IQ in 94–95

## T
tests
   Cloze 57
   comprehension 57
   eye movement monitoring 51
   for assessing reading and spelling 49
   hearing 41
   intelligence 63
   IQ 89, 94–95
   reading 7
   reading or spelling 94
   single word recognition 49
   spelling 39, 53
   standard performance 48
   Weschler 94
   Weschler intelligence scales 95
   word identification 49
transmission of information 1–2, 56

## V
verbal language
   primary processing centre of 25
   processing of 12
visual
   analysis 75
   analytic skills 63

Printed in the United Kingdom
by Lightning Source UK Ltd.
108226UKS00001B/487-561